Dash Diet Meal Plan

Weight Loss and Lower Blood Pressure in 30 Days

By:

William Devine

TABLE OF CONTENTS

This diet, coined as the 'Healthiest Diet', is designed to provide real-life solutions to high-blood pressure by suggesting a diet that merely regulates the intake of nutrients and not alter the common diet we're all used to. Dietary Approaches to Stop Hypertension or dash focuses on controlling the intake of sodium and fats to maintain the normal blood pressure of an individual. Dash is geared towards preparing a diet that makes satisfying meals, thus, preventing people from eating in-between meals, causing loss of control over food intake. Because it keeps people from hunger in-between meals, it ideally becomes more satisfying and less controlling.

The Dash diet teaches individuals to complete the whole dash diet program by starting with stocking up the kitchen with dash-friendly food, preparing dash-friendly recipes, and performing Dash-friendly exercises. Meal plans suggested by Dash usually contain ingredients high in fibre, calcium, magnesium and potassium. Dash diets go low on sodium and sugar and emphasize the need to eat green leafy vegetables and fruits.

Avocado dip, for instance, is one of the most famous Dash diets there is today, because of its very convenient and affordable Instructions. Avocado, a very rich source of monosaturated fat and lutein, (antioxidants that help protect vision), is among the many fruits that are highly-recommended for Dash diet. In this recipe, avocado has to be mashed and pitted, mixed with fat-free sour cream, onion and hot sauce. This dip shall be eaten with tortilla chips or sliced vegetables. From this dish, a person can get a total of 65 calories, 2 grams protein, 5 grams total fat, 4 grams carbohydrate, 172 milligrams potassium and 31 milligrams calcium. From this we can infer that a person is fed a considerable amount of necessary nutrients, essential for maintaining a well-balanced diet that's good for the heart.

In just fey days, a Dash diet follower will experience normal blood pressure, with fewer tendencies to eat in-between meals, the major culprit of weight gain. The Dash diet program also teaches individuals to determine the right amount of food intake, the necessary exercise to perform according to age and activity level. Dash educates and motivates --- one of the very important reasons why people find it easy to stick to the diet. Also, the diet does not require us to give up anything significant in our usual diet, instead, it helps us create a process of adjusting to little changes so we can successfully help ourselves.

Making a lifestyle change is an effort. It is a long-term commitment which one has to make for good health.

Making smaller changes will bring in faster results than making dramatic changes all at once and losing the commitment along the way.

WHAT IS A DASH DIET?

DASH stands for Dietary Approach to Stop Hypertension. DASH diet has been clinically proven to reduce blood pressure within 2 weeks in individuals following the diet. It is not only known to help manage the blood pressure but is also designed for weight loss programs, helps to prevent heart diseases, stroke, diabetes and some forms of cancer.

Diet plays a major role in both developing high blood pressure and also in lowering it. Food is our body's fuel. If you take a minute and think about it, consuming a poor diet is very similar to pumping leaded gas into a car that runs on unleaded. The engine will still start but it will run rough and over time will simply stop running because of carbon build up. Loading our bodies up with salt, sugar and saturated fat has the same impact.

The DASH diet plan works for two reasons. Firstly it is made up of foods rich in vitamins, minerals, fiber and antioxidants that lower pressure and reverse damage to the blood vessels. Secondly, and just as important, it replaces the junk that caused the problem in the first place.

It does take commitment to the diet to make it work and that will take some planning on your part particularly for meals you eat out. However, compare that bit of work to the drudgery and discomfort of blood pressure medication and I think you will agree that it is worth the effort.

Following the DASH diet plan, coupled with a bit of daily exercise and relaxation techniques, can drop your blood pressure reading by 20 points in less than two weeks. Give it a try. Your heart will thank you.

WHO SHOULD FOLLOW A DASH EATING PLAN?

In fact, a DASH eating plan can be a part of any healthy eating plan. Not only, will it help lower blood pressure but it will offer additional heart health benefits including lowering LDL cholesterol and inflammation.

HOW DOES THE DASH EATING PLAN WORK?

The diet consists of foods that are low in sodium and consists of a variety of foods that are rich in nutrients like potassium, calcium and magnesium are known to help lower blood pressure. The diet is rich in fibre that again helps to lower blood pressure and knock off the extra pounds which will in-turn assist in lowering blood pressure.

BENEFITS OF DASH DIET

Keeping track of one's diet is a healthy way of living because it allows one to check on his medical status. Many popular dietary regimens can be followed, and one of them is the DASH diet.

Here are some health benefits of Dash Diet

It Reduces The Risk Of Developing Heart Disease

Thanks to the DASH diet's unique ability to lower and control blood pressure, following this diet can make a big difference in your body's resistance to heart disease. A study from 2010 indicated that the DASH diet may "substantially" lower an individual's risk for coronary heart disease, which researchers said could bring "great public health benefits, given the enormous and persistent burden of coronary heart disease."

This is likely because lowered blood pressure allows your heart to function more effectively and efficiently, but could be beneficial for even those who don't struggle with hypertension and still want to prevent the onset of heart disease.

It Protects You From Certain Cancers

Researchers have examined the correlation between the DASH diet and various types of cancer, and have uncovered a positive association relating to reduced salt intake and monitoring consumption of dietary fat. The diet is also low in red meat, which has been linked to cancers of the colon, rectum, esophagus, stomach, lung, prostate, and kidney.

The focus on fresh produce helps prevent a number of cancers, and the emphasis on low-fat dairy can also contribute to a decreased risk for colon cancer.

You'll Be Able To Prevent Diabetes

The DASH diet has proven effective in helping prevent insulin resistance, which is shown to be linked to high blood pressure and cardiovascular health risks. By helping dieters manage their sodium intake, eat more fiber and potassium, and maintain a healthy weight, the DASH eating plan helps those who are predisposed to diabetes avoid or delay the onset of this condition.

According to some studies, this impact is even greater when the DASH plan is implemented as a component of a more comprehensive healthy lifestyle – including diet, exercise, and weight control.

Healthy Weight Maintenance

Whether you're looking to lose weight or not, the DASH diet is a great option to ensure you can stick to your goal weight once you've reached it. You can follow a customized version of the DASH diet to achieve your weight loss goals, then stick to a higher calorie count to maintain your new weight – and with the healthy options included in this diet, you won't have to deal with any weight gain after working so hard to lose it.

The DASH plan provides plenty of protein without overloading on carbs, meaning you'll enjoy building muscle and boosting your metabolism while keeping yourself from ever feeling heavy. And it's not a short-term diet – this is a new, healthy lifestyle.

WHAT SHOULD YOU EAT ON A DASH EATING PLAN?

Unlike many other diets that restrict your calorie consumption, followers of the DASH diet are encouraged to stick to the recommended daily intake for their age and activity level. The foods included in this eating plan are readily available for most people in the US, which is something researchers took into account when creating this diet – to ensure the public would be able to adopt the plan easily and successfully.

Fruits

Potassium is important for lowering blood pressure because it helps balance the electrolytes in our bodies. In fact, eating two bananas every day for two weeks proved in a study to lower blood pressure by 10 per cent – due to the fruit's high potassium content. However, tons of other fruits can give you some extra potassium to help keep your blood pressure healthy – citrus fruits, like oranges, lemons, limes, and grapefruits, are full of vitamins and minerals, and one avocado contains almost 700 mg of potassium.

The L-citrulline found in watermelon helps the body create L-arginine, an amino acid that improves circulation. Studies have shown that increased amounts of L-citrulline can even keep pre-hypertension from progressing to full blown hypertension – which is a significant risk factor for heart attacks and strokes.

Anthocyanins have also proven to provide significant protection against high blood pressure – and can be found in darker colored foods like blueberries, raspberries, strawberries, cranberries, blood oranges, and black currants. These flavonoids seem to have a beneficial effect on both blood vessels and blood flow, according to research.

Salt Substitutes

If you're someone who adds a lot of salt to your food to enhance the flavour, you'll need to find some other options that won't increase your sodium intake. Using acidic flavourings like lemon or lime juice or even vinegar can bring out the savoriness of your foods, and you can try chopped fresh or dried herbs, garlic, or salt-free seasoning blends to spice up your meals in a DASH friendly way.

Poultry, Fish, And Other Lean Meats

Full of B vitamins, vitamin E, magnesium, iron, zinc, and protein, lean meat is a healthy addition to your DASH diet. Focus on cuts that have a lower fat content – boneless, skinless chicken breasts, turkey cutlets, round steaks and roasts, and 90-97% lean ground meat.

Fish is also an important part of maintaining a DASH diet, particularly cold-water fish like tuna, mackerel, sardines, and salmon. With plenty of monounsaturated and polyunsaturated fats, including omega-3 fatty acids, this kind of fish is an important ally in your 🗌uest for a healthy cardiovascular system.

Whole Grains

While processed grains are sugary and contribute to a number of health issues, whole grains actually help reduce your risk of high blood pressure. Packed with fiber, whole grains will help keep you feeling full – so you won't need to snack on processed, unhealthy foods in between meals.

You'll also benefit from an increased intake of potassium, which has proven to help lower blood pressure. Whole grains also decrease your body's risk of resistance to insulin, and reduces damage to your blood vessels.

Vegetables

Research has shown that eating a high-fiber diet can lead to significant reductions in blood pressure – so the DASH diet encourages four to six servings of vegetables daily. You can easily increase the fiber in your diet by increasing your intake of vegetables – and you should aim to eat a variety of different colored produce every day.

Dairy

With tons of potassium and magnesium, low fat or non fat dairy can dramatically reduce your risk of developing high blood pressure. In addition to being fortified with calcium and rich in protein, dairy is a great heart-healthy food that should be included in any DASH eating plan.

If you're not concerned with weight management, you can indulge in whole fat dairy – but watch your portions and ensure you're not overeating.

Legumes, Seeds, And Nuts

Nuts are also full of valuable omega-3s, as well as protein and other heart healthy substances like fiber, unsaturated fats, and L-arginine. Legumes, including beans, lentils, and peas, also provide a hefty amount of magnesium and potassium, as well as protein and fiber. They also contain folate, which prevents the build-up of homocysteine – an amino acid which can raise your risk for heart attack and stroke.

To make this diet work even better here are some additional tips:-

- Stress can raise blood pressure even if the diet is healthy. Hence, stress management techniques like meditation, yoga, etc will help keep the blood pressure under check.
- Poor sleep increases blood pressure. So, 7-8 hours of sound sleep will help in keeping the blood pressure in control.
- Reducing alcohol intake may help reduce blood pressure. Hence, keep the alcohol intake under check.
- Aerobic exercise along with DASH diet works faster in lowering blood pressure.
- Read food labels to choose products that are lower in sodium.
- If you are someone who smokes, then quitting it would help lower blood pressure.
- Take your medication as prescribed.
- Limit the salt intake to 1 teaspoon a day.

Here are some common perceptions about the DASH diet, including what is—and what isn't—true.

The DASH Diet is Unapproachable.

Many equate healthy eating, particularly lower-sodium eating such as DASH, with the idea that all meals have to be cooked from scratch. This is overwhelming for many (myself included), but there are plenty of tricks and tips to help you. First, understand that "whole foods" doesn't exclusively mean fresh produce. Take advantage of time-saving, minimally processed foods like unseasoned frozen vegetables and no-salt-added canned veggies.

Two additional shortcuts that can easily be worked into a DASH diet plan are meal prepping and batch cooking—both of which are important for quick, healthy eating. Meal prepping doesn't have to mean cooking a full meal, either. It's just preparing components that can be used to toss together a quick meal—like baking chicken breasts, roasting vegetables, and cooking a whole grain like quinoa. You can also minimize time spent in the kitchen by buying weekly salad greens, bags of pre-cut veggies, and prepping produce at the start of the week.

The DASH Diet is Only for People With High Blood Pressure.

The DASH diet was created when researchers were looking for ways to effectively reduce hypertension, but this was over 20 years ago! Though it's still often marketed as a treatment for high blood pressure, the DASH eating plan is really an ideal way to eat for overall health, weight maintenance, and chronic disease prevention. In fact, studies suggest that DASH lowers risk for heart disease, type 2 diabetes and metabolic syndrome, and some cancers.

Also, people with high blood pressure aren't the only ones who need to worry about sodium intake. Data suggests that 90 percent of Americans exceed sodium's max limit (3500mg) daily. Regularly going over this amount takes a toll on your body—even healthy bodies—over time.

DASH is a "Diet" That You Follow Intermittently.

Perhaps the biggest thing that holds people back from following DASH is approaching it with an "all-or-nothing" attitude. However, DASH does not fall under the common "diet" approach of following an eating plan for a few weeks and then returning to your old way of eating. After all, no one's diet is perfect. Like the Mediterranean Diet, the DASH diet is best viewed as a healthy way of living and eating. Making small, gradual changes in your food choices—and food quality—can help you form healthier habits for life.

"Low-Sodium" and "No-Salt" are the DASH Diet's Sole Focus.

Sodium reduction is part of the DASH equation, but it's not the only focus. Eating by DASH recommendations also increases your intake of potassium, calcium, magnesium and fiber—all nutrients that play a role in cardiovascular health, as well as the prevention of other chronic diseases. It's thought to be the combination of increasing your intake of these nutrients and decreasing your intake of added sugar, salt, sodium and unhealthy fats that leads to lower blood pressure and a laundry list of other long-term health benefits.

Also, reducing sodium doesn't restrict you to boring, bland food, nor does it mean you have to toss out the salt shaker. Yes, reducing the amount of salt you use and choosing lower-sodium products are key, but opting for fresh foods or whole foods instead of boxed, canned, and ready-to-heat items makes a big enough impact. Experiment with spices and herbs, and use a little salt to enhance flavor. Salt should never be the sole flavoring or seasoning in any in dish.

HOW CAN I GET STARTED?

Since the DASH plan focuses primarily on plant-based foods, it's easy to incorporate this diet into your lifestyle by simply increasing your consumption of fruits and vegetables – along with portions of low and non-fat dairy, lean meats, poultry, and fish, plenty of whole grains, and a variety of healthy fats. However, if you're an inexperienced chef, you'll need to get used to spending some more time in the kitchen and develop some cooking skills to make the most of this eating plan.

This diet is very filling and easy to follow – so stock up on approved DASH plan foods and use these recipes to inspire your adventures in the kitchen. Hopefully, you'll discover some new favorite ingredients and learn interesting methods to prepare your food. The more you practice cooking DASH-style, the more you'll be able to come up with your own ways of creating healthier versions of classic recipes.

DASH DIET TIPS

Here are some tips to get you started

Choose low-fat dairy products

- Low-fat dairy products include 1% or skim (nonfat) milk, light yogurt, and 2% cheese. If you are currently eating or drinking high-fat dairy products, try the next step down. For example, if you drink whole milk, try 2% milk. If you drink 2% milk, try 1% milk.
- Order your favorite coffee beverage with non-fat or skim milk. This one small change can have a positive impact on your diet and health. Choosing low-fat dairy products helps to decrease the saturated fat ("bad fat") in your diet and increases important nutrients like calcium, magnesium, and potassium. Dairy products are naturally low in sodium too!
- But if your healthcare team has told you to limit potassium and phosphorus in your diet, then dairy products will need to be limited. Discuss your options with a dietitian.

Choose fruits and vegetables with intense color

The brighter or darker the fruit or vegetable, generally the more nutrients it contains.

Understand portions and serving sizes

For example, 1 cup of dry cereal or raw veggies are both equal to the size of a baseball; 1/2 cup of cooked pasta is the size of a computer mouse; and 3 ounces of cooked poultry, fish or meat should be the size of a deck of cards. Keep a measuring cup handy when preparing meals and snacks.

Drink more water

If you're trying to cut down on alcohol or reduce your intake of sugary fruit juices or sodas, this is a great way to keep yourself hydrated and less likely to indulge in some of those unhealthy alternatives. Water is important when you've upped your intake of fiber, so you can avoid the discomfort of constipation. You'll also be retaining less water as a result of lowered sodium consumption.

You can also consume additional water in the form of tea – another healthy alternative to sugary beverages or alcohol. Green tea is especially great for a healthy diet as it will speed up your metabolism and reduces your risk of developing cardiovascular disease. This is a perfect way to get more water and enjoy some other health benefits, as well.

Heart-healthy substitution

Instead of high-fat beef and other meats, choose lean meat, chicken, turkey, fish, tofu, low-sodium canned or dried beans such as lentils, chickpeas or kidney beans.

Instead of fatty, salty or sugary snacks like crackers, chips, cookies and candy, choose berries, grapes, fat-free yogurt, reduced-fat whole grain crackers, baked tortilla chips or plain popcorn.

Keep an eye on your blood pressure

This is especially key if you're not DASH dieting to lose weight. By regularly checking your blood pressure, you'll be able to track your progress and feel good about the results – giving you a bit of extra motivation to stick to your diet and lifestyle program to keep achieving greater health and wellness. It's exciting to see those numbers dropping, so give yourself the chance to celebrate.

Change gradually

To successfully adopt a healthier lifestyle, it's always a good idea to make small changes one step at a time rather than introducing a large, dramatic change. This way, you'll hardly notice each individual step – and you'll be much more likely to stay committed to your new, healthier lifestyle.

Think about what you already eat, and look for opportunities to incorporate DASH diet foods whenever you can. Focus more on vegetables instead of building your meal around meats or pastas. Eat fruit instead of desserts, or switch out your morning cup of orange juice for an actual orange, instead.

With a little Instructions, eating DASH-style can be second nature – and easy to keep up over time. Dried fruit or chopped veggies are easy to pack and bring with you for 🗌uick snacks at the office or on the go, so there's no excuse for straying from this healthy eating plan.

Read food labels

- The Nutrition Info label is your guide to what is inside all processed or packaged foods.
- Low sodium foods have ≤ less than 140 mg of sodium per serving, and
- Very low sodium products have ≤ less than 35 milligrams sodium per serving.

Day 1

Breakfast

Southwest Tofu Scramble

Prep Time 10 minutes
Cook Time 20 minutes
Total Time 30 minutes
Servings:2

Ingredients

SCRAMBLE

- 8 ounces extra-firm tofu
- 1-2 Tbsp olive oil
- 1/4 red onion (thinly sliced)
- 1/2 red pepper (thinly sliced)
- 2 cups kale (loosely chopped)

SAUCE

- 1/2 tsp sea salt
- 1/2 tsp garlic powder
- 1/2 tsp cumin powder

- 1/4 tsp chili powder
- Water (to thin)
- 1/4 tsp turmeric (optional)

FOR SERVING (optional)

- Salsa
- Cilantro
- Hot Sauce
- Breakfast potatoes, toast, and/or fruit

Instructions

- Pat tofu dry and roll in a clean, absorbent towel with something heavy on top, such as a cast-iron skillet, for 15 minutes.
- While tofu is draining, prepare sauce by adding dry spices to a small bowl and adding enough water to make a pourable sauce. Set aside.
- Prep veggies and warm a large skillet over medium heat. Once hot, add olive oil and the onion and red pepper. Season with a pinch each salt and pepper and stir. Cook until softened - about 5 minutes.
- Add kale, season with a bit more salt and pepper, and cover to steam for 2 minutes.
- In the meantime, unwrap tofu and use a fork to crumble into bite-sized pieces.
- Use a spatula to move the veggies to one side of the pan and add tofu. Sauté for 2 minutes, then

add sauce, pouring it mostly over the tofu and a little over the veggies. Stir immediately, evenly distributing the sauce. Cook for another 5-7 minutes until tofu is slightly browned.

- Serve immediately with the breakfast potatoes, toast, or fruit. I like to add more flavor with salsa, hot sauce, and/or fresh cilantro. Alternatively, freeze for up to 1 month and reheat on the stovetop or in the microwave.

Nutrition Info

Calories: 252
Fat: 19g Saturated
Fat: 3g Sodium: 516mg
Carbohydrates: 12.7g
Fiber: 3g
Sugar: 2.5g
Protein: 12g

Lunch

Tuna Salad and Spinach Sandwiches

Total Time: 10 min
Serves 4

Ingredients:

- One 6.4-ounce pouch light tuna packed in water
- 1/2 medium cucumber, peeled, seeded, and diced
- 1/2 small red onion, peeled and diced (about 1/4 cup)
- 2 ribs celery, diced
- 1/2 teaspoon dill weed
- 2 tablespoons olive oil
- Juice of one lemon
- 1/2 teaspoon salt-free seasoning blend
- 1/4 teaspoon freshly ground black pepper
- 8 slices 100% whole wheat sandwich bread
- 1 cup fresh baby spinach

Instructions

- Combine the tuna, cucumber, onion, celery, and dill weed. Drizzle with the olive oil and lemon juice, and stir. Season with salt-free seasoning blend and pepper. Make the sandwich with 1/2 cup tuna salad and 1/4 cup baby spinach leaves. Press down to compact the tuna and the spinach.

Note: This recipe will make 2 cups of tuna that will keep in the fridge for 3 days, long enough for more meals!

Nutrition Info

Calories: 194
Sodium: 450 milligrams
Potassium: 410 milligrams
Magnesium: 79 milligrams
Calcium: 81 milligrams

Dinner

Oven Roasted Turkey Breast

Prep time 5 mins
Cook time 1 hour 30 mins
Total time 1 hour 35 mins
Serve: 6

Ingredients

- 1 boneless turkey breast 2-3 pounds
- 1-2 tablespoons olive oil
- ½ teaspoon garlic powder
- 1 teaspoon minced dry onion
- 1 teaspoon seasoned salt
- 1 teaspoon smoked paprika
- ½ teaspoon pepper
- ½ teaspoon parsley flakes
- ½ teaspoon basil

Instructions

- Thaw turkey breast completely in the fridge
- Preheat oven to 350 and set out roasting pan or heavy deep oven proof dish
- Combine all seasonings in a small bowl and mix well
- Coat turkey with olive oil and rub in the spice mixture
- Place in baking pan on top of 3 or 4 aluminum foil balls
- Cook at 350 degrees for 90 minutes until internal temperature is 165-170 degrees
- Remove from oven and cover with foil, allow to rest 20-30 minutes before slicing

Nutrition Info

Calories 60
Total Fat 1.5g
Saturated Fat 0.5g
Trans Fat 0g
Cholesterol 25mg
Sodium 320mg
Total Carbohydrate 1g

Day 2

Breakfast

Pumpkin Breakfast Cookies

Prep Time: 10 minutes
Cook Time: 15 minutes
Total Time: 25 minutes
Serving: 12 cookies

Ingredients

- 1 cup (100g) rolled oats
- 1/2 cup (55g) coconut flakes
- 1/4 cup (40g) chia seeds (or flax seeds)
- 1/2 cup (125g) pumpkin puree
- 1/4 cup (80g) maple syrup
- 1/4 cup (75g) nut/seed butter of choice
- 1 tbsp pumpkin pie spice
- 1 tsp baking powder
- 1/4 tsp salt
- 1 tsp vanilla extract
- 1/4 cup (45g) chocolate chips (or chopped pecans would be good too!)

Instructions

- Preheat the oven to 350F.
- In a food processor, combine the oats, coconut, and chia seeds. Process until broken down into fine pieces but not quite flour.
- Add the pumpkin, nut butter, maple syrup, spice, baking powder, salt, and vanilla. Process until combined into a sticky dough.

- Add the chocolate chips, and process briefly until just combined.
- Roll into balls (about 1-1.5 tbsp of dough per cookie). Place on a baking sheet lined with parchment paper and press to flatten slightly.
- Bake for 15 minutes at 350F, or until the bottom edges are golden brown.
- Cool for at least 15 minutes.
- Enjoy!
- Keep leftovers in the fridge in an airtight container for up to a week, or freeze for longer storage.

Nutrition Info

Serving Size: 1 cookie
Calories: 145
Sugar: 7g
Fat: 7g
Saturated Fat: 3g
Carbohydrates: 16g

Lunch

Creamy Vegetable Lentil Soup

Prep Time: 10 minutes
Cook Time: 1 hour
Servings: 12 one cup

Total Time: 1 hour 10 min

Ingredients

- 1/4 cup olive oil
- 3 stalks celery or about 1 cup, chopped
- 3 medium carrots or about 1 cup, chopped
- 1 large white onion, diced
- 4 cloves garlic, minced
- 2 cups dry lentils
- 8 cups water
- 1 tablespoon reduced sodium vegetable bouillon
- 1 (14.5 ounce) can crushed tomatoes
- 2 teaspoons cumin
- 3 cups spinach, rinsed and roughly chopped
- ¼ cup chopped fresh basil or 1 tablespoon dried basil
- ½ cup white wine
- salt to taste
- ground black pepper to taste

Instructions

- In a large soup pot, heat oil over medium heat. Add carrots, celery and onions and cook, stirring occasionally for about 10 minutes or until the vegetables have softened. Stir in garlic and cook for another minute.

- Add lentils, water, tomatoes and cumin. Bring to a boil. Reduce heat to low, and simmer for about one hour or until lentils are tender.

- When lentils are tender, stir in spinach and basil, and cook until it wilts. Stir in wine, and season to taste with salt and pepper.

- For a creamy texture, remove about half of soup when cooled and puree in a blender. Add back to pot, garnish with basil, and enjoy!

Dinner

Turkey Swiss Roll-up

Prepare/Total: 10
Servings: 1

Ingredients

- 2 Romaine or Bibb Lettuce Leaf
- 3 Oz. Turkey Breast (sliced or shaved)
- 1 Oz. Swiss Cheese (sliced)
- 1 Tbsp. regular Mayo
- 2 Tbsp. Red Chopped Onion
- Black Pepper

Instructions

- Rinse and pat dry lettuce leaf, cut off stem, spread 1/2 tbsp. mayo on each leaf, spread red onions over mayo with black pepper, add 1.5 oz. turkey breast each leaf, add swiss cheese on each leaf, roll up lettuce length wise tucking in lettuce.

Nutrition Info

Servings Per Recipe: 1
Amount Per Serving
Calories: 295.4
Total Fat: 19.3 g
Cholesterol: 66.5 mg
Sodium: 1,009.2 mg
Total Carbs: 6.7 g
Dietary Fiber: 1.1 g
Protein: 23.2 g

Day 3

Breakfast

Banana Almond Smoothie

Prep Time: 3 mins
Cook Time: 2 mins
Total Time: 5
Serves: 2

Ingredients

- 1 medium to large frozen banana (break your bananas into one-inch chunks before freezing)
- 1 heaping spoonful of almond butter (or peanut butter)
- 2 spoonfuls flax seed
- ½ cup almond milk, yogurt or regular milk
- drizzle of honey, agave nectar or maple syrup
- tiny drop of almond extract (or vanilla extract, but the almond extract makes the smoothie taste almost like candy!)

Instructions

- Toss all the ingredients into a blender and blend until smooth.
- Pour into a glass and enjoy.

Notes

- Adapted from the New York Times Recipes for Health.
- Since this smoothie doesn't require any ice, just frozen banana.

Nutrition Info

Calories: 154.6

Total Fat: 7.7 g
Protein: 3.2 g
Sugars: 9.3 g

Lunch

Chicken Vegetable Soup

Prep Time 20 minutes
Cook Time 35 minutes
Total Time 55 minutes
Servings: 4

Ingredients

- 1 tablespoon butter
- 1/2 cup onion finely diced
- 2 carrots peeled, halved lengthwise and sliced
- 2 stalks celery thinly sliced
- 2 teaspoons minced garlic
- 3 cups cooked chicken shredded or cubed
- salt and pepper to taste
- 15 ounce can diced tomatoes do not drain
- 8 ounce can tomato sauce
- 1 teaspoon Italian seasoning
- 6 cups chicken broth
- 1 large Russet potato peeled and cut into 1/2 inch cubes
- 1/2 cup frozen corn

- 1/2 cup diced green beans fresh or frozen
- 2 tablespoons chopped fresh parsley

Instructions

- Melt the butter in a large pot over medium high heat. Add the onion, carrots and celery to the pot.
- Cook for 5-6 minutes or until softened. Add the garlic and cook for 30 seconds more. Season with salt and pepper to taste.
- Add the chicken, tomatoes, tomato sauce, Italian seasoning, chicken broth and potato to the pot; bring to a simmer.
- Cook for 20-25 minutes or until potatoes are tender. Taste and add salt and pepper as desired.
- Stir in the corn and green beans and cook for 5 minutes more. Sprinkle with parsley and serve.

Nutrition Info

Calories: 284kcal
Carbohydrates: 24g
Protein: 21g
Fat: 12g
Saturated Fat: 3g
Cholesterol: 58mg
Sodium: 762mg
Potassium: 1010mg

Dinner

Vegetable Stirfry over Quinoa

Prep Time: 15 mins
Cook Time: 15 mins
Total Time: 30 mins
Serving: 6

Ingredients

- 1 cup of carrots, julienned
- 1 red pepper, julienned
- 1 yellow pepper, julienned
- 1 head of broccoli, chopped
- 8 oz. of baby portobello mushrooms, quartered
- 1 zucchini, halved lengthwise and sliced
- 4 green onions, chopped
- 2 garlic cloves, minced
- 1 T.fresh ginger, minced
- 1/3 cup Kikkoman low sodium soy sauce
- 1/4 cup chicken stock
- 1 tsp. red pepper flakes
- 1 tsp. dry mustard
- 1 tsp. sugar
- 1 T. sesame oil
- 1 T. rice wine vinegar
- 1 T. flour

Instructions

- Chop up your vegetables.
- Heat wok or large skillet to medium high heat, add 2 T. of sesame oil, ginger, and garlic. Saute for 30 seconds, don't let the garlic burn.
- Add in the carrots, red pepper, and yellow pepper. Saute for 2-3 minutes.
- Add in the mushrooms, broccoli, and zucchini. Saute for 3-4 minutes, stirring occasionally.
- Cover and let sit for 6-8 minutes.
- In a small bowl, mix together low sodium soy sauce, chicken stock (or vegetable stock), red pepper flakes, dry mustard, sugar, sesame oil, rice wine vinegar. In another small bowl, mix 1 T. of flour and 1 T. of water together. Add to stirfry sauce mixture. (this will help thicken the sauce)
- Remove cover and add in stirfry sauce and green onions. Stir together. Put cover back on for one more minute and you are good to go. ??
- For the Quinoa, just follow the simple instructions on the package.
- Enjoy!

Nutrition Info

287 calories
10.1 g fat

37.7 g carbohydrates
11.7 g protein
93 mg cholesterol
621 mg sodium.

Day 4

Breakfast

Slow Cooker, Apple Cinnamon Steel-Cut Oatmeal

Prep Time: 10 minutes
Cook Time: 6 hours
Total Time: 6 hours 10 minutes
Servings: 7 (3/4-cup) servings

Ingredients

- 2 apples, peeled, cored, cut into 1/2-inch pieces (2-1/2 to 3 cups chopped)
- 1-1/2 cups fat-free milk (or substitute non-diary alternative like almond milk)
- 1-1/2 cups water
- 1 cup uncooked steel-cut oats
- 2 tablespoons brown sugar (or substitute maple syrup or other desired sweetener)
- 1-1/2 tablespoons butter, cut into 5-6 pieces (optional)
- 1/2 teaspoon cinnamon

- 1 tablespoon ground flax seed
- 1/4 teaspoon salt
- Optional garnishes: chopped nuts, raisins, maple syrup, additional milk or butter

Instructions

- Coat inside of 3-1/2 Quart (or larger) slow cooker with cooking spray. Add all ingredients (except optional toppings) to slow cooker. Stir, cover, and cook on low for approx. 7 hours (slow cooker times can vary). Spoon oatmeal into bowls; add optional toppings, if desired. Store leftovers in refrigerator. Freezes well.

- To reheat single servings: Put 1-cup cooked oatmeal in microwave proof bowl. Add 1/3 cup fat-free milk. Microwave on high for 1 minute; stir. Continue cooking for another minute, or until hot.

Note: Recipe can be doubled in 6-Quart or larger slow cooker. Increase cooking time 1 hour.

Nutrition Info

149 calories,
3.6g fat,
27.3g carbs,
3.9g fiber,

4.9g protein

Lunch

Healthy Everyday Rainbow Salad

Prep Time: 10 mins
Total Time: 10 mins
Serving: 1

Ingredients

For the Rainbow Salad

- 1 big handfuls of fresh spinach
- 1 big handful of de-stemmed and finely chopped kale
- raw grated beet (about 1 small beet)
- finely chopped red cabbage
- raw grated carrot (about 1 small carrot)
- peeled, chopped and roasted acorn squash
- finely chopped, steamed broccoli
- 1 tbsp each sunflower seeds and pumpkin seeds
- 1/4 of an avocado, diced
- dried kelp flakes

For the Sweet Ginger Miso Dressing

- 1/4 tbsp water
- big chunk of peeled, fresh ginger
- 3 tbsp tahini
- 2 tbsp pure maple syrup
- 2 tbsp miso paste
- 2 tbsp apple cider vinegar
- 1 tbsp soy sauce (or gluten-free tamari)

Instructions

- To make the salad dressing, blend all ingredients until smooth. If desired, add more water to adjust consistency. Season with salt and pepper, if desired.
- To assemble the salad, add everything to a bowl and top with the dressing.

Nutrition Info

Calories 35 Cal
Carbs5 g
Dietary Fiber4 g
Sugar1 g
Sodium68 mg
Potassium0 mg
Cholesterol0 mg

Dinner

Garlic Mashed Potatoes

Prep 10 m
Cook 25 m
Total Time: 35 m
Serves 8

Ingredients

- 2 pounds all-purpose red or gold potatoes, scrubbed and cut into large chunks
- 6 cloves garlic, peeled
- 1/4 cup olive oil
- 1 teaspoon salt-free seasoning blend
- 1/2 teaspoon freshly ground black pepper

Instructions

- Place the potato chunks and peeled garlic cloves in a large saucepan. Cover with cold water and bring to a boil.

- Reduce the heat and cook for about 25 minutes, or until the potatoes are tender when pierced with a fork.

- Remove from heat.

- Drain the cooking liquid off the potatoes, reserving 3/4 cup of the cooking liquid.

- Add the olive oil, salt-free seasoning blend, pepper, and reserved cooking liquid to the potatoes.

- Mash with a potato masher or large fork.

- Taste and season with more salt-free seasoning and pepper, if you like.

Nutrition Info

Calories: 145
Sodium: 7 milligrams
Potassium: 527 milligrams
Magnesium: 26 milligrams
Calcium: 16 milligrams
Fat: 7 grams
Saturated Fat: 1 gram
Cholesterol: 0 milligrams
Protein: 2 grams

Day 5

Breakfast

Mushroom Spinach Omelet

Prep Time: 3 mins

Cook Time: 15 mins
Total Time: 18 mins
Serving: 1 omelet

Ingredients

- 1 tablespoon olive oil
- 1/4 cup slice red onion
- 1 1/2 cup fresh spinach
- 5 baby bella mushrooms, sliced
- 1 oz goat cheese
- Cooking Spray
- 1 whole egg
- 2 egg whites
- green onions, diced (for optional garnish)

Instructions

- Heat a medium skillet to medium high heat. Add olive oil and red onions to the pan. Saute for 2-3 minutes until the onions are translucent.
- Add the sliced mushrooms to the pan, saute until the mushrooms are slightly browned. Approximately 4-5 minutes.
- Next add spinach to the pan. Saute until the spinach is wilted, about 2 minutes. Season with salt and pepper. Set aside.
- Heat a small skillet to medium heat. Spray with cooking spray.

- In a small bowl, add one whole egg and two egg whites. Whisk to mix.
- Add the egg mixture to the small skillet. Let the mixture sit for one minute. Gently take a spatula and work your way around the edges of the skillet. Then lift the skillet and tilt it down and around in a circular fashion so as to get the "runny" eggs in the center to cook along the edges you just cleaned. Continue this process for another minute.
- Add the mushroom spinach mixture to one side of the omelete top with crumbled goat cheese. Using your spatula, gently fold the other side of the omelet over the mushroom spinach side. Let cook for 30 seconds and gently transfer omelet to a plate. Top with green onions

Nutrition Info

Serving Size: 1 omelet
Calories: 412
Sugar: 8 g
Sodium: 332 mg
Fat: 29 g
Carbohydrates: 18 g
Fiber: 4 g
Protein: 25 g
Cholesterol: 199 mg

Lunch

Salmon Topper Stuffed Avocados

Prep Time 10 Min
Cook Time 5 Min
Total Time 15 Min

Ingredients

- 1 avocado, halved and pitted
- 4.5 oz. True North Salmon Toppers
- ¼ cup diced red bell pepper
- 1 tbsp. minced jalapeno
- ¼ cup cilantro leaves, roughly chopped
- 1 tbsp. lime juice
- Salt and pepper (to taste)

Instructions

- Scoop out some of the avocado from the pitted area to widen the "bowl" area. Place the scooped avocado into a medium-size mixing bowl. Mix with a fork.
- Add the True North Salmon Toppers, bell pepper, jalapeno, and cilantro to bowl. Pour lime juice over. Stir until everything is well mixed.

- Scoop the Salmon Topper mixture into the avocado bowls. Season to taste with salt and pepper.

Nutrition info

Calories 463 cal
Total Carbs 13.9grams
Fiber 7.5grams
Net Carbs 6.4grams
Protein 27grams
Fat 34.6 grams

Dinner

Easy Roasted Salmon

Prep: 5 min
Cook: 15 min
Total: 20 min
4 servings

Ingredients

- Four 6-ounce wild salmon fillets
- One lemon, cut into 4 wedges
- Freshly ground black pepper
- 1/4 cup minced fresh dill (from one small bunch)

- 4 cloves garlic, peeled and minced

Instructions

- Preheat oven to 400 F. Coat a glass baking dish with nonstick cooking spray. Place the salmon fillets in the baking dish.

- Squeeze juice from one wedge of lemon over each fillet.

- Sprinkle the salmon with black pepper, dill, and garlic.

- Bake until the salmon is opaque in the center, about 20 to 22 minutes.

Nutrition Info

Calories: 251
Sodium: 78 milligrams
Potassium: 894 milligrams
Magnesium: 53 milligrams
Calcium: 36 milligrams

Day 6

Breakfast

Pumpkin Pie Yogurt Parfait

Prep Time10 minutes
Total Time10 minutes
Servings 1

Ingredients

- 1/2 cup pumpkin puree exact amount depends on the size of your parfait glass
- 1/2 cup yogurt (Greek yogurt works especially well here)
- 2 Tbsp. pecans, chopped or granola
- 1/2 tsp. cinnamon
- 1/8 tsp. ground cloves
- 1 tsp. honey Optional- to taste

Instructions

- Mix the pumpkin with the pumpkin spices and half of the honey, to taste. I find pumpkin puree sweet enough on its own for me, but most people will probably want to sweeten it a little.
- Fill the parfait glass a little under a fourth of the way up with (around half of) the pumpkin puree mixture.
- If you're using pecans, toast them and sprinkle a thin layer of them over the layer of pumpkin puree. You can also use granola instead.

- Mix the yogurt with the rest of the honey, to taste.
- Cover the pecans or granola with a layer of yogurt, followed by a thin layer of pecans or granola, followed by the rest of the pumpkin puree.
- Add a dollop of yogurt on top, and garnish with more pecans or granola.
- Enjoy!

Nutrition Info

Calories: 343kcal
Carbohydrates: 26g
Protein: 8g
Fat: 25g
Saturated Fat: 4g

Lunch

Quinoa Meatless Balls

Prep Time: 30 minutes
Cook Time: 30 minutes
Total Time: 1 hour
Serving: 18 large meatballs

Ingredients

- ½ cup dry Quinoa, pre-rinsed
- 1 cup water
- 1 cup cooked green lentils, well drained
- ¼ cup diced red bell pepper
- ½ cup diced onion
- 2 cloves garlic, minced
- ½ cup gluten free bread crumbs or whole wheat panko bread crumbs (add additional bread crumbs if the meatballs need to be firmer and aren't holding together well)
- ¼ cup freshly grated parmesan
- 1 tablespoon freshly chopped flat parsley leaves
- 1 tablespoon freshly chopped oregano
- 1/2 teaspoon freshly ground black pepper
- Sea salt to taste
- ¼ teaspoon cayenne pepper
- 1 egg white (for vegan add 2-3 teaspoons water)
- 3 tablespoons olive oil

Instructions

- Add pre-rinsed Quinoa and water to a medium pot, cover, bring to a boil. Reduce heat to a simmer and continue cooking 15 minutes or until water is completely absorbed. In the meantime, in a large non-stick skillet add 1 tablespoon olive oil, heat to medium-low and sauté diced onions and bell pepper until tender about 4 minutes, add garlic, parsley and oregano and sauté one additional minute.

- Remove Quinoa from heat and allow to rest 10 minutes. Press down on Quinoa with a paper towel to remove any remaining water.
- In a large mixing bowl combine sautéed onion, garlic, parsley and oregano along with remaining ingredients, except oil. Use either a potato masher or fork and mash the ingredients until the lentils are well mashed. Using your hands, shape into 1 ½ " (meatless) meatballs, place in a large bowl, cover and refrigerate until chilled, about 2 hours.
- Add remaining 2 tablespoons oil to a large non-stick skillet, heat to medium-low and add Quinoa (meatless) meatballs. Brown meatballs, turn over and brown on the other side. Cook until browned and heated through, about 16 minutes. Remove from skillet and drain on a paper towel.
- If you plan to serve these (meatless) meatballs with marinara, add to the marinara sauce, gently turn to coat. Simmer until hot and serve over pasta.
- These are a perfect food to eat prior to working out as they provide complex carbohydrates for energy and protein for building muscles. When on hand, I'll have a few before a workout.
- TIP: For a vegan version, use vegan egg replacer or 1 tbsp of flaxmeal mixed with 3 tbsp

water rather than the 2-3 teaspoons straight water.

Nutrition Info

Calories: 291
Total Fat: 10 g
Saturated Fats: 2 g
Trans Fats: 0 g
Cholesterol: 3 mg
Sodium: 293 mg
Carbohydrates: 139g
Dietary fiber: 6 g

Dinner

Spicy Roasted Broccoli

Prep Time: 5 minutes
Cook Time: 15 minutes
Total Time: 20 minutes
Servings: 4 people

Ingredients:

- 1 1/4 pounds broccoli, large stems trimmed and cut into 2-inch pieces (about 8 cups)
- 4 tablespoons olive oil, divided
- 1/2 teaspoon salt-free seasoning blend

- 1/4 teaspoon freshly ground black pepper
- 4 cloves garlic, peeled and minced
- 1/4 teaspoon crushed red pepper flakes

Instructions

- Preheat the oven to 450 F.

- In a large bowl, toss together the broccoli and 2 tablespoons olive oil. Sprinkle with salt-free seasoning and pepper.
- Transfer to a rimmed baking sheet and bake for 15 minutes. Meanwhile, mix together 2 tablespoons olive oil, the garlic, and the red pepper flakes.
- After the broccoli has cooked 15 minutes, drizzle the garlic oil over the broccoli and shake the baking sheet to coat the broccoli.
- Return to the oven and continue baking until the broccoli starts to brown, about 8 to 10 more minutes.
- Serve hot.

Nutrition Info

Calories: 86
Calcium: 37 milligrams
Fat: 7 grams
Saturated Fat: 1 gram
Cholesterol: 0 milligrams

Carbohydrate: 5 grams
Protein: 2 grams

Day 7

Breakfast

Easy Buckwheat Crepes

Prep Time 10 minutes
Cook Time 15 minutes
Total Time 25 minutes
Servings: 3

Ingredients

CREPES

- 1 cup un-toasted (raw) buckwheat flour (*not kasha or Bob's Red Mill brand - we recommend grinding your own flour from buckwheat groats - see notes!)
- 3/4 Tbsp flaxseed meal
- 1 3/4 cups light (canned) coconut milk (we found almond milk and lighter, less fatty milks to promote sticking to the pan)
- 1 pinch sea salt
- 1 Tbsp avocado or melted coconut oil (plus a bit more for cooking // or use nonstick pan)

- 1/8th tsp ground cinnamon (optional // omit for savory)
- sweetener (optional // to taste // I used a dash of stevia // omit for savory or unsweetened)

FILLINGS optional

- Compote
- Nut Butter
- Coconut Whipped Cream
- Granola
- Cinnamon Baked Apples

Instructions

- To a blender or mixing bowl, add buckwheat flour flaxseed meal, light (canned) coconut milk, salt, avocado oil, cinnamon (omit for savory), and sweetener of choice (omit for savory or unsweetened).
- Pulse in blender or whisk in mixing bowl to combine. The batter should be pourable but not watery. If too thin, add a bit more buckwheat flour. If too thick, thin with more dairy-free milk.

- Heat a cast-iron or nonstick skillet over medium heat. (Non-stick is typically best for crepes, but I used a seasoned cast-iron skillet and it worked well, too). Once hot, add a little oil and spread into an even layer. Let the oil heat until hot - when you flick a little water onto the pan, it should crackle and evaporate almost immediately.

- Add ~1/4 cup (60 ml) batter. Let cook until the top appears bubbly and the edges are dry (similar to pancakes). Then carefully flip and cook for 2-3 minutes more on the other side. Turn heat down if cooking too quickly.

- Repeat until all crepes are prepared. We didn't find we needed to add any more oil after the first crepe. Keep warm between layers of parchment paper or on a plate under a towel.
- Serve as is with a little vegan butter, nut butter, maple syrup, compote, or other fillings or choice! My preferred is vegan butter, berries, maple syrup, and banana. But these would also be delicious with coconut whipped cream, Cinnamon Baked Apples, fresh fruit (e.g. berries or bananas), or granola.
- Best when fresh, but you can store leftovers sealed in the refrigerator up to 3 days. To freeze, layer between pieces of parchment paper (to prevent sticking) and freeze. Then store in a freezer-safe container up to 1 month. To reheat, warm in a 350-degree F (176C) oven or microwave until hot.

Nutrition Info

Calories: 71
Fat: 3g
Saturated fat: 3g
Sodium: 28mg
Potassium: 62mg
Carbohydrates: 8g Fiber: 1g
Protein: 1g
Calcium: 0.6% Iron: 2.5%

Lunch

Vegetable Sushi

Prep: 1 hr
Cook: 20 min
Total: 1 hr 20 min
Servings: 20 rolls

Ingredients

For the rice:

- 3 cups short-grain Japanese rice, rinsed
- 1/3 cup rice vinegar
- 3 tablespoons sugar
- Salt

For the rolls:

- 10 nori sheets (dried seaweed), halved
- Sesame seeds, for sprinkling
- 1 cucumber
- 1 avocado
- 1 plum tomato, seeded
- 1 small red onion
- 20 asparagus spears, trimmed and blanched
- Wasabi paste, for spreading and serving
- 1 romaine lettuce heart
- Pickled ginger, for serving

Instructions

- Make the rice. Combine the rice and 3 1/4 cups water in a rice cooker and cook according to the manufacturer's instructions. A rice cooker is the best way to get perfect sticky-firm rice, but if you don't have one, just use a saucepan. Fold in the vinegar. Combine the vinegar, sugar and 1 teaspoon salt in a saucepan over medium heat, stirring to dissolve the sugar. Transfer the cooked rice to a large wooden bowl (traditionally, a wooden tub). Drizzle a quarter of the vinegar mixture over a wooden spoon or spatula onto the rice. Fold the rice gently with the spoon to cool it and break up any clumps; be careful not to smash the grains. Fold in the remaining vinegar mixture and let the rice sit 5 minutes. Spread the rice.

- Cover a bamboo sushi mat with plastic wrap. Place a half nori sheet rough-side up on the mat. Moisten your hands and scoop a handful of rice, slightly larger than a lemon, onto the nori. Press the rice to spread it evenly up to the edges of the nori, moistening your fingers as you go. Sprinkle with sesame seeds.

- Prepare the vegetables. Peel the cucumber and slice into matchsticks. (Morimoto cuts the entire cucumber into a paper-thin sheet, then quickly slices it into strips-but he's had some practice.) Thinly slice the avocado, tomato and red onion; peel the tough ends of the asparagus. Add the filling. Carefully flip over the nori so it's rice-side down on the mat with the short end facing you. Spread a bit of wasabi paste in a line about one-third of the way up the nori-it's spicy, so use it sparingly. Arrange a few pieces each of lettuce, cucumber, avocado, tomato and onion in a tight pile in the lower third of the sheet. It's OK if the vegetables hang over the edges of the nori. Roll the sushi. Roll the sushi away from you with your hands, tucking in the vegetables as you go. Remove the mat from under the roll and place it on top. Press the roll into a compact rectangular log, using the mat to help you. Slice the roll. Cut the sushi roll into 4 to 6 pieces. Repeat with the remaining nori, rice and vegetables. Serve with pickled ginger and more wasabi.

Nutrition Info

Calories 143 calorie
Total Fat 1 grams
Saturated Fat 0 grams

Dinner

Spicy Roasted Broccoli

Prep Time: 5 minutes
Cook Time: 15 minutes
Total Time: 20 minutes
Servings: 4 people

Ingredients

- 1 1/4 pounds broccoli, large stems trimmed and cut into 2-inch pieces (about 8 cups)
- 4 tablespoons olive oil, divided
- 1/2 teaspoon salt-free seasoning blend
- 1/4 teaspoon freshly ground black pepper
- 4 cloves garlic, peeled and minced
- 1/4 teaspoon crushed red pepper flakes

Instructions:

- Preheat the oven to 450 F.
- In a large bowl, toss together the broccoli and 2 tablespoons olive oil. Sprinkle with salt-free seasoning and pepper.
- Transfer to a rimmed baking sheet and bake for 15 minutes. Meanwhile, mix together 2 tablespoons olive oil, the garlic, and the red pepper flakes.
- After the broccoli has cooked 15 minutes, drizzle the garlic oil over the broccoli and shake the baking sheet to coat the broccoli.
- Return to the oven and continue baking until the broccoli starts to brown, about 8 to 10 more minutes.
- Serve hot.

Nutrition Info

Calories: 86
Calcium: 37 milligrams
Fat: 7 grams
Saturated Fat: 1 gram
Cholesterol: 0 milligrams
Carbohydrate: 5 grams
Protein: 2 grams

Day 8

Breakfast

Ezekiel Bread French Toast

Prep Time 5 minutes
Cook Time 15 minutes
Total Time 20 minutes
Servings 2 Servings

Ingredients

- 4 Slices Ezekiel Bread
- 2 Eggs
- 1/2 Cup Coconut Milk or Unsweetened Almond Milk lite or silk
- 2 Tbsp Coconut Sugar
- 1 pkt Stevia
- 1 tsp vanilla
- Pinch Salt
- Cinnamon

Instructions

- Mix everything except for the Ezekiel bread together in a large mixing bowl.

- Dip each slice of bread in the mixture, covering both sides with liquid.

- Cook each side in a skillet for about 5 minutes, or until lightly browned.

- Add syrup and enjoy!

Nutrition Info

Calories 335 kcal

Lunch

Salmon Poke Bowl

Prep Time: 5 minutes
Cook Time: 20 mins
Total Time: 25 min
2 servings

Ingredients

for 1 serving

- 1 cup sushi rice (200 g)
- 1 cup water, plus more for rinsing (240 mL)
- 3 tablespoons rice vinegar
- 1 ½ teaspoons sugar
- ½ teaspoon salt
- 8 oz wild-caught, sushi-grade salmon fillet (225 g)

- 2 tablespoons soy sauce
- 2 tablespoons lemon juice
- ½ avocado, thinly sliced
- ½ cucumber, halved lengthwise and thinly sliced
- 2 tablespoons pickled ginger
- 1 green onion, thinly sliced
- 5 small sheets nori
- ¼ teaspoon toasted sesame seeds
- ¼ teaspoon black sesame seeds

Instructions

- Add the rice to a fine mesh strainer and submerge in a bowl filled with water. Shake the rice a few times to remove excess starch.
- Transfer the rice to a medium pot and add 1 cup (240 ml) of water. Cover the pot and bring to a boil over medium-high heat. Once boiling, reduce the heat to medium-low and simmer for 10 minutes. Remove the pan from the heat and let stand for 15 minutes.
- Remove the lid and fluff the rice with a fork or rice paddle. Transfer the rice to a large bowl.
- Mix together the rice vinegar, sugar, and salt and pour over the rice while still hot. Gently fold the rice to incorporate. Cover and set aside until ready to assemble the bowl.
- Using a very sharp knife, gently slice the salmon fillet into ½-inch (1 cm) cubes. It may

be easier to slice if you place the salmon in the freezer for a few minutes to help it firm up.

- Just before assembly, place the salmon in a bowl and season with the soy sauce and lemon juice.
- To assemble, place a few spoonfuls of rice into a medium bowl (use any leftover rice for another poke bowl or sushi). Top the rice with the seasoned salmon, avocado, cucumber, ginger, green onions, nori sheets, toasted sesame seeds, and black sesame seeds.
- Enjoy!

Nutrition Info

Calories: 771 cal
Fat52.54g
Saturated fat10.14g
Trans fat
Carbs24.33g

Dinner

Apple-Cherry Pork Medallions

Prep/Total Time: 30 min.
Serving: 4 serves

Ingredients

- 1 pork tenderloin (1 pound)
- 1 teaspoon minced fresh rosemary or 1/4 teaspoon dried rosemary, crushed
- 1 teaspoon minced fresh thyme or 1/4 teaspoon dried thyme
- 1/2 teaspoon celery salt
- 1 tablespoon olive oil
- 1 large apple, sliced
- 2/3 cup unsweetened apple juice
- 3 tablespoons dried tart cherries
- 1 tablespoon honey
- 1 tablespoon cider vinegar
- 1 package (8.8 ounces) ready-to-serve brown rice

Instructions

- Cut tenderloin crosswise into 12 slices; sprinkle with rosemary, thyme and celery salt. In a large nonstick skillet, heat oil over medium-high heat. Brown pork on both sides; remove from pan.
- In same skillet, combine apple, apple juice, cherries, honey and vinegar. Bring to a boil, stirring to loosen browned bits from pan. Reduce heat; simmer, uncovered, 3-4 minutes or just until apple is tender.
- Return pork to pan, turning to coat with sauce; cook, covered, 3-4 minutes or until pork is

tender. Meanwhile, prepare rice according to package Instructions; serve with pork mixture.

Nutrition Info

349 calories
9g fat (2g saturated fat)
64mg cholesterol
179mg sodium
37g carbohydrate (16g sugars, 4g fiber)
25g protein.

Day 9

Breakfast

Blueberry Banana Muffins

Prep time 20 Minutes
Cook time 25 Minutes
Serving: 12 large muffins

Ingredients

- 3/4 cup (190 mL) mashed ripe banana (about 2 medium)
- 3/4 cup + 2 tablespoons (220 mL) unsweetened almond milk
- 1 teaspoon apple cider vinegar

- 1/4 cup (60 mL) pure maple syrup
- 1 teaspoon pure vanilla extract
- 1/4 cup (60 mL) coconut oil, melted
- 2 cups (280 g) white spelt flour
- 4 to 6 tablespoons (40 to 60 g) coconut sugar or natural cane sugar*
- 2 teaspoons baking powder
- 1 1/2 teaspoons cinnamon
- 1/2 teaspoon fine grain sea salt
- 1/2 teaspoon baking soda
- 1/2 cup (50 g) walnut halves, chopped (optional)
- 1 1/4 cups (160 g) frozen or fresh blueberries**

Instructions

Preheat oven to 350°F and grease a muffin tin.

- In a medium bowl, mash bananas and measure out 3/4 cup. If you have any leftover mashed banana you can freeze it for a smoothie.
- Place mashed banana into medium bowl along with the milk, vinegar, maple syrup, and vanilla. No need to stir it yet.
- Melt the coconut oil in a small pot over low heat. Set aside.
- In a large bowl, mix together the dry ingredients (flour, sugar, baking powder, cinnamon, salt, and baking soda).

- Stir coconut oil into the wet mixture. Pour wet ingredients onto the dry ingredients and stir until just combined. Do not overmix as spelt is a fragile little flour.
- Gently fold in the walnuts and then the blueberries, being sure not to overmix as this can result in dense muffins.
- Spoon a heaping 1/4 cup of batter into each muffin tin, filling each tin about 3/4 full (they will be almost full, but this is normal). I like to press a few extra blueberries on top of each so they look pretty after baking.
- Bake at 350°F for 23 to 27 minutes until a toothpick comes out clean. I baked them for 25 minutes.
- ·Cool in pan for 5 to 8 minutes and then transfer muffins to a cooling rack and cool for another 15 minutes.

Nutrition Info

Calories: 229.6
Total Fat: 9.5 g
Sugars: 0.6 g
Saturated Fat: 0.8 g

Lunch

Pesto-flavoured Spelt Salad

Prep : 10 min
Cooking : 35 min
Savings: 4

Ingredients

- 2/3 cup spelt berries
- 23 leaves fresh basil
- 1/2 clove garlic
- 3 tbsp pine nuts
- 4 tsp Parmesan cheese
- 1/4 cup extra virgin olive oil
- 1 pinch salt [optional]
- ground pepper to taste [optional]

Before you start

Please note: Depending on the type of spelt berries used, they may require soaking at least 4 h before cooking.

A blender or food processor will be very useful to make the pesto sauce.

Instructions

- Put the spelt berries in a pot, cover with water then bring to a boil. Add a little salt, cover, and simmer until the berries are cooked, about 35 min. Drain and set aside.

- Meanwhile, combine the garlic, pine nuts and basil in a food processor or a blender and finely chop. Add the grated cheese and olive oil, then mix until a creamy, but thick consistency is achieved.
- Toss the mixture with the cooked spelt. Adjust the seasoning, then serve hot or at room temperature.

Nutrition Info

Calories ?270 cal
Fat :0 g
Cholesterol :0 mg

Dinner

Chocolate Banana Cake

Total: 55 mins
Prep: 15 mins
Cook: 40 mins
Serving: 12 to 16 Servings

Ingredients

- 2 cups all-purpose flour

- 1/2 cup Splenda Brown Sugar Blend
- 1/4 cup unsweetened cocoa powder
- 1/2 teaspoon baking soda
- 1 large ripe banana, mashed (1/2 cup)
- 3/4 cup soy milk
- 1/4 cup canola oil
- 1 large egg
- 1 egg white
- 1 tablespoon lemon juice
- 1 teaspoon vanilla extract
- 1/2 cup semisweet dark chocolate chips

Instructions

- Preheat oven to 350 F.

- Coat an 11- by 7-inch brownie pan with nonstick spray.

- Whisk together flour, brown sugar blend, cocoa, and baking soda in large bowl.

- In another bowl, whisk together the bananas, soy milk, oil, egg, egg white, lemon juice, and vanilla.

- Make a hole in the middle of the flour mixture, and pour in the soy milk mixture and chocolate chips.

- With a wooden spoon, stir the ingredients together until blended. Spoon the batter into the pan.

- Bake about 25 minutes until the center of the cake springs back when pressed lightly with fingertips.

Nutrition Info

Calories: 150
Sodium: 52 milligrams
Potassium: 119 milligrams
Magnesium: 19 milligrams
Calcium: 23 milligrams
Fat: 4 grams

Day 10

Breakfast

Healthy Breakfast Cookies

Prep: 10 minutes
Cook: 15 minutes
Servings: 12 cookies

Ingredients

- 1 cup creamy peanut butter (or other nut butter)
- 1/4 cup honey
- 1 teaspoon vanilla extract
- 2 medium ripe bananas, mashed
- 1/2 teaspoon salt
- 1 teaspoon ground cinnamon
- 2 1/4 cups Quick oats
- 1/2 cup dried cranberries or raisins
- 2/3 cup chopped nuts, such as almonds, walnuts or pistachios

Instructions

- Preheat the oven to 325°F. Line a baking sheet with parchment paper or a Silpat.

- In the bowl of a stand mixer fitted with the paddle attachment, beat together the peanut butter, honey, vanilla extract, mashed bananas, salt and cinnamon.

- Add the oats, dried cranberries and nuts and mix until combined. Scoop about 1/4-cup mounds of the cookie dough onto the baking sheet, flattening each cookie slightly. (The cookies will not spread while baking, so you can space them relatively close together.)

- Bake the cookies for 14 to 16 minutes until they're golden brown but still soft. Remove the cookies from the oven then allow them to cool for 5 minutes on the baking sheet before transferring them to a rack to cool completely.

Nutrition Info

Calories: 55 (or 35 calories each, if you use a mini cookie scoop)
Fat: 2.5g.
Carbs: 6g.
Protein: 1.5g.
Added sugars: 0 grams.
Fiber: 1g.

Lunch

Three-Bean Kale Saute with Brown Rice

Prep Time: 5 minutes
Cook Time: 15 minutes
Total Time: 20 min
Servings: 8 servings

Ingredients

- 1 cup black beans
- 1 cup red kidney beans

- 1 cup white beans
- 4 tbsp extra-virgin olive oil, divided
- 1/4 tsp sea salt
- 1/4 tsp black pepper
- 1 tsp crushed red-pepper flakes
- 4 garlic cloves, smashed
- 1/2 cup low-sodium vegetable broth
- 1 lb kale, stems and leaves coarsely chopped
- 2 tbsp red wine vinegar
- 4 cups cooked brown rice, prepared according to Instructions

Instructions

- Cook the beans according to Instructions on label or use canned beans. Drain and rinse the beans, then drain again.
- In a mixing bowl, combine beans with 2 tablespoons of the oil, salt, pepper and red-pepper flakes and toss thoroughly.
- In a large sauté pan, heat the remaining 2 tablespoons oil over medium-high heat. Add the garlic and cook until soft but not browned.
- Turn the heat up to high, add the broth and kale and stir to combine. Cover and cook for 3 to 4 minutes.
- Add the beans, stir and cook covered for an additional 3 to 4 minutes or until the liquid is evaporated.

- Remove from the heat, toss with the vinegar, top each serving with 1/2 cup brown rice and serve immediately, accompanied by a salad.

Nutrotion Info

Calories: 277 cal

Dinner

Curried Cauliflower Steaks with Red Rice & Tzatziki

Prep 30 m
Total Time: 1 h
4 servings

Ingredients

Tzatziki

- ¾ cup nonfat plain Greek yogurt
- ¼ cup sour cream
- 1 tablespoon lemon juice
- 1 clove garlic, minced
- ½ teaspoon kosher salt
- ½ medium cucumber, seeded and grated
- 1 cup red rice or brown basmati rice
- ? cup extra-virgin olive oil

- 1 tablespoon lemon juice
- 2 teaspoons curry powder
- ½ teaspoon kosher salt
- 2 medium heads cauliflower
- 2 tablespoons chopped fresh cilantro

Instructions

- To prepare tzatziki: Whisk yogurt, sour cream, lemon juice, garlic and salt in a medium bowl until smooth. Fold in cucumber. Refrigerate. To prepare rice & cauliflower: Preheat oven to 450°F. Line a large rimmed baking sheet with foil. Prepare rice according to package Instructions. Keep warm. Meanwhile, whisk oil, lemon juice, curry powder and salt in a small bowl. Remove any outer leaves from cauliflower, but keep stems intact. Place on a cutting board, stem-side down. Using a large chef's knife, cut two 1-inch-thick slices from the center of each head to make 4 cauliflower "steaks." Cut enough of the remaining cauliflower into ¾-inch florets to get 4 cups. Place the steaks and florets in a single layer on the prepared baking sheet. Brush both sides with the curry mixture. Roast, gently turning halfway through, until the florets are lightly browned and the cauliflower-steak stems are tender, 30 to 35 minutes. Refrigerate the florets and 6 tablespoons tzatziki for another use (see

Tip, below). Divide the rice among 4 plates and top each portion with a cauliflower steak, ¼ cup tzatziki and a sprinkle of cilantro.

- To make ahead: Refrigerate tzatziki (Step 1) for up to 5 days; refrigerate roasted cauliflower florets for up to 3 days.

Tips: Turn leftovers into a Curried Cauliflower Salad for lunch: Combine 6 Tbsp. leftover tzatziki with 1 sliced scallion and ½ tsp. curry powder. Chop the reserved roasted cauliflower florets; stir into the sauce with 1/2 cup diced cucumber and ¼ cup rinsed canned chickpeas. Serve garnished with cilantro, with a 6-inch whole-wheat pita.

Nutrition info

410 calories
21 g fat(4 g sat)
7 g fiber
49 g carbohydrates
10 g protein
113 mcg folate
6 mg cholesterol
5 g sugars

Day 11

Muesli Scones

Serves:16scones

Ingredients

- 2 cups blanched almond flour (not almond meal)
- ½ teaspoon celtic sea salt
- ½ teaspoon baking soda
- ¼ cup dried cranberries
- ¼ cup dried apricots, cut into ¼-inch pieces
- ¼ cup sunflower seeds
- ¼ cup raw sesame seeds
- ¼ cup pistachios, coarsely chopped
- 1 large egg, size does matter as dough will not hold together with a small or medium egg
- 2 tablespoons agave nectar or honey

Instructions

- In a large bowl, combine almond flour, salt and soda
- Stir in dried fruit, seeds and nuts
- In a small bowl combine egg and agave
- Stir wet ingredients into dry
- Use your hands to form dough

- Shape dough into a 6½ x 6½ square that is about ¾-inch thick
- Cut dough into 16 squares
- Bake at 350°F on a parchment paper lined baking sheet for 10-12 minutes
- Serve

Nutrition Info

Calories: 123.324 cal
2.8g Fat Total
1.5g Saturated Fat
1.3g Fibre
3.1g Protein

Lunch

Veggie & Hummus Sandwich

Prep/Total 10 m
1 serving

Ingredients

- 2 slices whole-grain bread
- 3 tablespoons hummus
- Sabra Supremely Spicy Hummus 10 Oz
- $2.79 for 1 itemThru 02/10
- ¼ avocado, mashed

- ½ cup mixed salad greens
- ¼ medium red bell pepper, sliced
- ¼ cup sliced cucumber
- ¼ cup shredded carrot

Instructions

- Spread one slice of bread with hummus and the other with avocado. Fill the sandwich with greens, bell pepper, cucumber and carrot. Slice in half and serve.

- To make ahead: Refrigerate sandwich for up to 4 hours.

Nutrition info

325 calories;
14 g fat(2 g sat);
12 g fiber;
40 g carbohydrates;
13 g protein;
171 mcg folate;
0 cholesterol; 7 g

Dinner

Turkey Burgers

Prep: 15 m
Cook: 15 m
Ready In: 30 m
12 servings

Ingredients

- 3 pounds ground turkey
- 1/4 cup seasoned bread crumbs
- 1/4 cup finely diced onion
- 2 egg whites, lightly beaten
- 1/4 cup chopped fresh parsley
- 1 clove garlic, peeled and minced
- 1 teaspoon salt
- 1/4 teaspoon ground black pepper

Instructions

- In a large bowl, mix ground turkey, seasoned bread crumbs, onion, egg whites, parsley, garlic, salt, and pepper. Form into 12 patties.
- Cook the patties in a medium skillet over medium heat, turning once, to an internal temperature of 180 degrees F (85 degrees C).

Nutrition Info

183 calories
9.5 g fat
2.3 g carbohydrates

20.9 g protein

90 mg cholesterol

354 mg sodium.

Day 12

Breakfast

Summer Breakfast Quinoa Bowls

Prep Time:5 minutes
Cook Time:20 minutes
Total Time:25 minutes
2 servings

Ingredients:

- 1 small peach, sliced
- 1/3 cup uncooked Quinoa, rinsed well
- 2/3 + 3/4 cup almond milk
- 1/2 tsp vanilla extract
- 2 tsp brown sugar (or sweetener of your choice)
- 12 raspberries
- 14 blueberries
- 2 teaspoons local honey

Instructions

- In sauce pan cook combine Quinoa and 2/3 cup almond milk, vanilla and brown sugar.
- Cook on medium heat and bring to boil for five minutes.
- Lower the heat to low and cover.
- Cook for 15 to 20 minutes, or until easily fluffs with a fork.
- Meanwhile, heat a grill pan and spray with oil.
- Grill the peaches to bring out their sweetness 2 to 3 minutes; set aside.
- Warm the remaining almond milk.
- Divide the cooked Quinoa between 2 bowls then pour in warmed almond milk.
- Top with peaches, raspberries and blueberries and drizzle each with 1 teaspoon of honey.

Nutrition Info

Calories: 180 calories
Total Fat: 4g
Saturated Fat: 0g
Cholesterol: 0mg
Sodium: 136mg
Carbohydrates: 36g
Fiber: 4g

Lunch

Quinoa Unstuffed Peppers

Prep/Total Time: 30 min.
4 servings

Ingredients

- 1-1/2 cups vegetable stock
- 3/4 cup Quinoa, rinsed
- 1 pound Italian turkey sausage links, casings removed
- 1 medium sweet red pepper, chopped
- 1 medium green pepper, chopped
- 3/4 cup chopped sweet onion
- 1 garlic clove, minced
- 1/4 teaspoon garam masala
- 1/4 teaspoon pepper
- 1/8 teaspoon salt

Instructions

- In a small saucepan, bring stock to a boil. Add Quinoa. Reduce heat; simmer, covered, until liquid is absorbed, 12-15 minutes. Remove from heat.
- In a large skillet, cook and crumble sausage with peppers and onion over medium-high heat until no longer pink, 8-10 minutes. Add garlic and seasonings; cook and stir 1 minute. Stir in Quinoa. Freeze option: Place cooled Quinoa mixture in freezer containers. To use, partially

thaw in refrigerator overnight. Microwave, covered, on high in a microwave-safe dish until heated through, stirring occasionally.

Nutrition Info

1 cup: 261 calories,
9g fat (2g saturated fat),
42mg cholesterol,
760mg sodium,
28g carbohydrate (3g sugars, 4g fiber),
17g protein.

Dinner

Mediterranean Chicken Kabobs

Prep Time: 25 minutes
Cook Time: 10 minutes
Servings: 6

Ingredients

- 1-2 teaspoon chopped garlic
- 2 tablespoons finely chopped fresh or 2 teaspoons dried rosemary leaves
- 1 tablespoon finely chopped fresh or 1 teaspoon dried oregano leaves
- 1 teaspoon salt

- 1/2 teaspoon pepper
- 1/4 cup lemon juice
- 4-5 tablespoons olive oil
- 1 1/2 lb boneless skinless chicken breasts, cut into 1-inch pieces

Optional:

- 1 large red bell pepper, cut into 1-inch pieces
- 1 large red onion, cut into 1-inch wedges

Instructions

- In mix together garlic, rosemary, oregano, salt, pepper, lemon juice, and olive oil. Add chicken and coat well. Pour into a large resealable ziplock bag. Seal and refrigerate overnight to marinate.
- Heat gas or charcoal grill.
- Remove chicken from marinade; discard marinade. Slide chicken pieces onto wood or metal skewers (optional: alternately thread chicken, bell pepper and onion, leaving space between pieces)
- Place skewers on grill over medium-high heat. Cover grill; cook 8 to 10 minutes, turning occasionally, cook until chicken is no longer pink in center and vegetables are tender.

Nutrition Info

Calories: 114.1 kcal
Protein: 4.1 g
Carbs: 1.0 g
Fat: 10.6 g
Fiber: 0.1 g
Sugar: 0.2 g
Sodium: 397.3 mg

Day 13

Breakfast

Cinnamon Toast Breakfast Quinoa

Prep Time: 3 mins
Cook Time: 7 mins
Total Time: 10 minutes
1 serving

Ingredients

Breakfast Quinoa

- Heaping 2 tablespoons chopped raw pecans
- 1 ½ teaspoons coconut oil
- ½ teaspoon ground cinnamon, plus more for sprinkling on top
- Tiny pinch of salt

- 1 cup pre-cooked 🞎uinoa* (either chilled or warm from cooking—both will work)
- 1 tablespoon maple syrup, more if desired

Toppings and optional accompaniments

- 1 tablespoon chopped dried cherries or dried cranberries
- Hemp seeds, chia seeds or flax seeds (optional), for serving
- Milk or yogurt of choice (totally optional), for serving

Instructions

- First, toast the pecans before we add the remaining ingredients. To do so, warm the pecans in a small saucepan (use a larger saucepan if you are making multiple servings) over medium heat, shimmying the pan often, until the pecans smell fragrant and toasty, about 4 to 6 minutes.
- Add the coconut oil, cinnamon and salt to the pot. While stirring constantly, cook until the cinnamon is fragrant, about 15 seconds.
- Add the 🞎uinoa to the pot and stir to combine. Cook, while stirring constantly, just until the 🞎uinoa is warmed through, about a minute or so. Remove the pan from heat and stir in the maple syrup.

- Transfer the mixture to a bowl and top with dried fruit and a hefty sprinkle of hemp seeds, if using. Top with a light sprinkle of cinnamon. Serve promptly, with additional maple syrup and milk or yogurt on the side, if you'd like.

Nutrition Info

Serving Size 1 cup cooked (185 g)
Calories 222
Calories from Fat 36
Total Fat 4g 6%
Saturated Fat 0g 0%

Lunch

Floridian Grilled Veggie Sandwich

Prep Time: 10 minutes
Cook Time: 10 minutes
Total Time: 20 minutes

Ingredients

- 1 small onion (sliced)
- 1 ½ tablespoons lite mayonnaise
- ¼ cup fat free cheese (crumbled)
- ½ cup red bell pepper (sliced)
- Baby Spinach

- 1 clove of garlic
- ½ tablespoon lemon juice
- 2 tablespoons olive oil
- ½ zucchini (sliced)
- ½ yellow squash (sliced)
- 2 slices focaccia bread

Instructions

- Mix mayonnaise, lemon juice, and garlic in a bowl and keep in the fridge.
- Preheat the grill over high heat.
- Spray the vegetables with olive oil and grease the rack of the grill.
- Grill all the vegetables for 3-5 minutes. The peppers can take a bit longer. Take away from the grill and keep aside.
- Spread lite mayonnaise equally on bread slices, sprinkle feta cheese and put on the grill (cheese side up). Cover with a lid for 2 minutes.
- Remove from the grill and layer with the vegetables.
- Open faced grilled sandwich is ready to serve.

Nutrition Info

Calories: 240
Fat: 14 g
Carb: 24 g
Protein: 7 g

Dinner

White Beans & Bow Ties

Prep/Total Time: 25 min.
Makes 4 servings

Ingredients

- 2-1/2 cups uncooked whole wheat bow tie pasta (about 6 ounces)
- 1 tablespoon olive oil
- 1 medium zucchini, sliced
- 2 garlic cloves, minced
- 2 large tomatoes, chopped (about 2-1/2 cups)
- 1 can (15 ounces) cannellini beans, rinsed and drained
- 1 can (2-1/4 ounces) sliced ripe olives, drained
- 3/4 teaspoon freshly ground pepper
- 1/2 cup crumbled feta cheese

Instructions

- Cook pasta according to package Instructions. Drain, reserving 1/2 cup pasta water.
- Meanwhile, in a large skillet, heat oil over medium-high heat; saute zucchini until crisp-tender, 2-4 minutes. Add garlic; cook and stir

30 seconds. Stir in tomatoes, beans, olives and pepper; bring to a boil. Reduce heat; simmer, uncovered, until tomatoes are softened, 3-5 minutes, stirring occasionally.

- Stir in pasta and enough pasta water to moisten as desired. Stir in cheese.

Tip: Boost protein in meatless pasta dishes by using whole wheat noodles, adding white beans or stirring in a little cheese—or all three!

Nutrition Info

1-1/2 cups: 348 calories, 9g fat (2g saturated fat), 8mg cholesterol, 394mg sodium, 52g carbohydrate (4g sugars, 11g fiber), 15g protein.

Day 14

Breakfast

Mushroom-Shallot Frittata

Total Time:30 minutes
4 servings

Ingredients

- 4 shallots, finely chopped

- 1/2 lb mushrooms, finely chopped
- 2 tsp fresh chopped parsley
- 1 tsp thyme
- 3 eggs
- 5 large egg whites
- 1 tbsp fat free half and half (or milk)
- 1/4 cup fresh grated Pecorino Romano
- 1 tbsp butter
- salt and fresh pepper

Instructions

- Preheat oven to 350°.
- Heat butter in a large skillet over medium heat.
- Stir in shallots and saute until golden, about 5 minutes. Add chopped mushroom, thyme, parsley, salt and pepper.
- In a medium bowl whisk eggs, egg whites, parmesan, half and half, salt, and pepper.
- Add eggs to the skillet making sure eggs cover all the mushrooms. When the edges begin to set (about 2 minutes) move the skillet to oven.
- Cook about 15 minutes, or until frittata is completely cooked.
- Serve warm, cut into 4 equal wedges.

Nutrition Info

Calories: 132 calories
Total Fat: 7.5g

Saturated

Vegetarian Quinoa Chili

Prep Time: 10 minutes
Cook Time: 45 minutes
Total Time: 55 minutes
Serving: Serves 10-12

Ingredients

- 1/2 cup Quinoa, rinsed
- 1 cup water
- 1 tablespoon olive oil
- 1 small onion, chopped
- 3 cloves garlic, minced
- 1 jalapeno pepper, diced
- 1 large carrot, peeled and chopped
- 2 celery stalks, chopped
- 1 green bell pepper, chopped
- 1 red bell pepper, chopped
- 1 medium zucchini, chopped
- 2 (15 ounce) cans black beans, drained and rinsed
- 1 (15 ounce) can red kidney beans, drained and rinsed
- 3 (15 ounce) cans diced tomatoes

- 1 (15 ounce) can tomato sauce
- 2-3 tablespoons chili powder, depending on your taste (we used 3)
- 1 tablespoon ground cumin
- Salt and black pepper, to taste
- Optional toppings: green onions, avocado slices, cheese, sour cream, Greek yogurt, chips, crackers, etc.

Instructions

- In a medium sauce pan, combine the Quinoa and water. Cook over medium heat until water is absorbed, about 15 minutes. Set aside.
- In a large pot, heat the olive oil over high heat. Add the onion and cook until tender, about 5 minutes. Stir in garlic, jalapeño, carrot, celery, peppers, and zucchini. Cook until vegetables are tender, about 10 minutes.
- Add the black beans, kidney beans, tomatoes, and tomato sauce. Stir in the cooked Quinoa. Season with chili powder, cumin, salt, and black pepper. Simmer chili on low for about 30 minutes. Serve warm.

Nutrition Info

Calories: 256 cal

Dinner

Chicken with Orzo Salad (Mediterranean)

Prep 40 m
Total Time: 40 m
4 servings

Ingredients

- 2 skinless, boneless chicken breasts (8 ounces each), halved
- 3 tablespoons extra-virgin olive oil, divided
- 1 teaspoon lemon zest
- ½ teaspoon salt, divided
- ½ teaspoon ground pepper, divided
- ¾ cup whole-wheat orzo
- 2 cups thinly sliced baby spinach
- 1 cup chopped cucumber
- 1 cup chopped tomato
- ¼ cup chopped red onion
- ¼ cup crumbled feta cheese
- 2 tablespoons chopped Kalamata olives
- 2 tablespoons lemon juice
- 1 clove garlic, grated
- 2 teaspoons chopped fresh oregano

Instructions

- Preheat oven to 425°F. Brush chicken with 1 tablespoon oil and sprinkle with lemon zest and ¼ teaspoon each salt and pepper. Place in a baking dish. Bake until an instant-read thermometer inserted in the thickest part registers 165°F, 25 to 30 minutes. Meanwhile, bring a quart of water to a boil in a medium saucepan over high heat. Add orzo and cook for 8 minutes. Add spinach and cook for 1 minute more. Drain and rinse with cold water. Drain well and transfer to a large bowl. Add cucumber, tomato, onion, feta and olives. Stir to combine. Whisk the remaining 2 tablespoons oil, lemon juice, garlic, oregano and the remaining ¼ teaspoon each salt and pepper in a small bowl. Stir all but 1 tablespoon of the dressing into the orzo mixture. Drizzle the remaining dressing over the chicken and serve with the salad.

Nutrition info

Serving size: ½ chicken breast & 1 cup orzo salad
Per serving: 402 calories; 7 g fat(4 g sat); 6 g fiber; 28 g carbohydrates; 32 g protein

Day 15

Breakfast

Peanut Butter Overnight Oats

Prep Time 6 hours 5 minutes
Total Time 6 hours 5 minutes
Servings:

Ingredients

OATS

- 1/2 cup unsweetened plain almond milk (DIY recipe)
- 3/4 Tbsp chia seeds
- 2 Tbsp natural salted peanut butter or almond butter (creamy or crunchy)
- 1 Tbsp maple syrup (or sub coconut sugar, organic brown sugar, or stevia to taste)
- 1/2 cup gluten-free rolled oats

TOPPINGS optional

- Sliced banana, strawberries, or raspberries
- Flaxseed meal or additional chia seed
- Granola

Instructions

- To a mason jar or small bowl, add almond milk, chia seeds, peanut butter, and maple syrup (or other sweetener) and stir with a spoon to combine. The peanut butter doesn't need to be completely mixed with the almond milk (doing so leaves swirls of peanut butter to enjoy the next day).

- Add oats and stir a few more times. Then press down with a spoon to ensure all oats have been moistened and are immersed in almond milk.
- Cover securely with a lid or plastic wrap and set in the refrigerator overnight (or for at least 6 hours).
- The next day, open and enjoy as is or garnish with desired toppings (see options above).
- Overnight oats will keep in the refrigerator for up to 2 days, though best within the first 12-24 hours.

Nutrition info

Calories: 454
Fat: 23.9g
Saturated fat: 2g
Sodium: 162mg
Carbohydrates: 50.9g
Fiber: 12g
Sugar: 14.9g
Protein: 14.6g

Lunch

Grilled Flatbread Pizza

Prep Time: 3 hr
Cook Time: 6 min
Servings: 4 small pizzas (4-8 servings)

Ingredients

For the Flatbread:

- 1 1/2 cups (350 grams) warm water
- 2 teaspoons (16 grams) honey
- 1 teaspoon (4 grams) active dry yeast
- 4 cups (460 grams) all-purpose flour
- 1 teaspoon (6 grams) kosher salt
- 2 tablespoons (27 grams) olive oil

For Grilling and Topping the Pizzas:

- Olive oil
- Toppings of your choosing

Instructions

- Mix the water and honey in the bowl of a stand
  mixer. Sprinkle the yeast on top and set aside
  for 10-15 minutes, until foamy.

- Add two cups of the flour and gently mix until thoroughly incorporated. Cover with plastic wrap and set aside in a warm place for an hour.

- Add the salt, oil, and remaining two cups of flour, and mix with a dough hook for 5-7 minutes to knead the dough. Coat the dough in oil, place it in a clean bowl, and cover it with plastic wrap. Set the dough in a warm place to rise for about an hour, or until approximately doubled in size.

- Punch the dough down with floured hands and divide it into four discs. Place the discs on a lightly floured baking sheet, cover with a clean kitchen towel, and set aside to rise in a warm place for 30 minutes.

- When you are ready to cook, preheat the grill to high. Flour your hands and spread each dough disc into a thin oval, allowing a little thickness around the edges. Brush olive oil onto the top of each dough oval. Carefully place pizza dough on the grill, oiled side down. Close the grill and let cook for 2-3 minutes.

- Brush the tops of the dough with oil, carefully flip, and layer on your desired toppings.

- Close the grill and cook for 2-3 more minutes, or until the cheese is melted. Remove from the grill, slice, and serve hot.

Nutrition Info

Calories 250
Calories from Fat 99 (39.6%)
Total Fat 11g
Saturated fat 4.5g
Cholesterol 35mg
Sodium 680mg

Dinner

Lemon-Herb Salmon with Caponata & Farro

Prep Time 20 min
Cook Time: 30 m
Total Time: 50 m
4 servings

Ingredients

- 2 cups water
- 1/2 cup farro
- 1 medium eggplant, cut into 1 inch cubes
- 1 red bell pepper, cut into 1-inch pieces
- 1 summer squash, cut into 1-inch pieces

- 1 small onion, cut into 1-inch pieces
- 1½ cups cherry tomatoes
- 3 tablespoons extra-virgin olive oil
- ¾ teaspoon salt, divided
- ½ teaspoon ground pepper, divided
- 2 tablespoons capers, rinsed and chopped
- 1 tablespoon red-wine vinegar
- 2 teaspoons honey
- 1¼ pounds wild salmon (see Tips), cut into 4 portions
- 1 teaspoon lemon zest
- ½ teaspoon Italian seasoning
- Lemon wedges for serving

Instructions

- Position racks in upper and lower thirds of oven; preheat to 450°F. Line 2 rimmed baking sheets with foil and coat with cooking spray. Bring water and farro to a boil in a saucepan. Reduce heat to low, cover and simmer until just tender, about 30 minutes.
- Drain if necessary. Meanwhile, toss eggplant, bell pepper, squash, onion and tomatoes with oil, ½ teaspoon salt and ¼ teaspoon pepper in a large bowl. Divide between the prepared baking sheets.
- Roast on the upper and lower racks, stirring once halfway, until the vegetables are tender and starting to brown, about 25 minutes.

Return them to the bowl. Stir in capers, vinegar and honey.

- Season salmon with lemon zest, Italian seasoning and the remaining ¼ teaspoon each salt and pepper and place on one of the baking sheets.
- Roast on the lower rack until just cooked through, 6 to 12 minutes, depending on thickness. Serve the salmon with the farro, vegetable caponata and lemon wedges.

Nutrition Info

Per serving: 450 calories; 17 g fat(3 g sat); 8 g fiber; 41 g carbohydrates; 35 g protein; 77 mcg folate; 66 mg cholesterol; 12 g sugars; 3 g added sugars; 1,738

Day 16

Breakfast

Green Breakfast Smoothie

Prep Time: 5 minutes
Cook Time: 0 minutes
Total Time: 5 minutes
Servings: 1 serving

Ingredients

- 1 small banana, frozen
- 1/2 cup pineapple
- 1 handful kale or spinach
- 1/4 avocado
- 1 tsp chia seeds
- 2 tbsp plant-based protein powder (optional)
- 1/4 cup orange juice
- 1/2 cup almond milk

Instructions

- Blend all ingredients in a high-speed blender until smooth.

- Pour into a glass and serve.
- Notes

- Add in your favourite superfoods to this smoothie like turmeric, spirulina and maca powder.

- Substitute frozen cauliflower for the frozen banana if you'd like a low-sugar smoothie option.

- Use unflavoured or vanilla protein powder.

Nutrition Info

Serving Size: 1 smoothie
Calories: 333
Sugar: 29g
Fat: 14g
Saturated Fat: 2g
Carbohydrates: 52g
Fiber: 10g
Protein: 5g

Lunch

Cobb Salad

Prep 20 m
Cook 30 m
Ready In 50 m
6 servings

Ingredients

- 6 slices bacon
- 3 eggs
- 1 head iceberg lettuce, shredded
- 3 cups chopped, cooked chicken meat
- 2 tomatoes, seeded and chopped
- 3/4 cup blue cheese, crumbled
- 1 avocado - peeled, pitted and diced
- 3 green onions, chopped

- 1 (8 ounce) bottle Ranch-style salad dressing

Instructions

- Place eggs in a saucepan and cover completely with cold water. Bring water to a boil. Cover, remove from heat, and let eggs stand in hot water for 10 to 12 minutes. Remove from hot water, cool, peel and chop.
- Place bacon in a large, deep skillet. Cook over medium high heat until evenly brown. Drain, crumble and set aside.
- Divide shredded lettuce among individual plates.
- Evenly divide and arrange chicken, eggs, tomatoes, blue cheese, bacon, avocado and green onions in a row on top of the lettuce.
- Drizzle with your favorite dressing and enjoy.

Nutrition Info

525 calories
39.9 g fat
10.2 g carbohydrates
31.7 g protein
179 mg cholesterol
915 mg sodium.

Dinner

Chicken Chili with Sweet Potatoes

Prep Time: 10 min
Cook Time: 12 min
Total Time: 22 minutes
5 servings

Ingredients

- 2 tablespoons extra-virgin olive oil
- 1 large onion, chopped
- 3 cloves garlic, minced
- 2 cups cubed sweet potato (½-inch)
- 1 medium green bell pepper, chopped
- 2 tablespoons chili powder
- 2 teaspoons ground cumin
- 1 teaspoon dried oregano
- 1 15-ounce can low-sodium cannellini beans, rinsed
- 2 cups low-sodium chicken broth or homemade chicken stock
- 1 cup frozen corn
- 2 cups cubed cooked chicken (½-inch; about 10 ounces)
- ¾ teaspoon salt
- Great Value Salt, 26 oz
- ¼ teaspoon ground pepper
- Sour cream, avocado and/or cilantro for garnish

Instructions

- Heat oil in a large pot over medium-high heat. Add onion, garlic, sweet potato and bell pepper; cook, stirring occasionally, until the vegetables are slightly softened, 5 to 6 minutes.
- Stir in chili powder, cumin and oregano and cook, stirring, until fragrant, 1 minute. Add beans and broth (or stock) and bring to a boil.
- Reduce heat, partially cover and simmer gently for 15 minutes. Increase heat to medium-high and stir in corn; cook 1 minute.
- Add chicken and cook until heated through, 1 to 2 minutes more.
- Remove from heat. Stir in salt and pepper.
- Serve topped with sour cream, avocado and/or cilantro, if desired.

Nutrition info

324 calories
10 g fat(2 g sat)
8 g fiber
35 g carbohydrates
26 g protein
29 mcg folate
48 mg cholesterol

5 g sugars;

Day 17

Breakfast

Fruit Pizza

Prep Time: 1 hour, 10 minutes
Total Time: 2 hours
Serving: serves 10-12

Ingredients:

Sugar Cookie Crust

- 1/2 cup (115g) unsalted butter, softened to room temperature
- 3/4 cup (150g) granulated sugar
- 1 large egg, at room temperature
- 1 teaspoon vanilla extract
- 1 and 1/2 cups (190g) spoon & leveled all-purpose flour
- 1/4 teaspoon salt
- 1 teaspoon baking powder
- 1/2 teaspoon baking soda
- 1 and 1/2 teaspoons cornstarch

Topping

- 8 oz (224g) full-fat cream cheese, softened to room temperature
- 1/4 cup (60g) unsalted butter, softened to room temperature
- 2 cups (240g) confectioners' sugar
- 1-2 Tablespoons (15-30ml) cream or milk
- 1 teaspoon vanilla extract
- assorted sliced fresh fruit

Instructions

Make the crust

- In a large bowl using a hand-held mixer or stand mixer fitted with a paddle attachment, cream the softened butter for about 1 minute on medium speed. Get it nice and smooth, then add the sugar and beat on medium speed until fluffy and light in color. Beat in egg and vanilla. Scrape down the sides as needed.
- In a medium bowl, whisk the flour, salt, baking powder, baking soda, and cornstarch together. With the mixer running on low speed, slowly add the dry ingredients to the wet ingredients. Once completely combined, cover the dough tightly and chill in the refrigerator for 30 minutes and up to 1 day. Without chilling, your cookie dough may spread over the sides of the pan.

- Preheat oven to 350°F (177°C). Grease a 12-inch pizza pan. Remove chilled cookie dough from the refrigerator and press onto the pizza pan in an even flat circle, as pictured above. Bake for 18-20 minutes or until the edges are very lightly browned. Overbaking will lend a hard crust. Allow crust to cool completely before decorating. I put the crust in the refrigerator after 10 minutes of cooling at room temperature - this sped up the process.
- I usually use this time (as the crust cools) to chop the fruit.

Make the frosting

- In a medium bowl using a handheld or stand mixer fitted with a paddle or whisk attachment, beat the cream cheese and butter together on medium speed until smooth, about 2 minutes. Add the confectioners' sugar and 1 Tbsp cream. Beat for 2 minutes. Add the vanilla and 1 more Tbsp cream if needed to thin out. Beat for 1 minute. Spread in a thick layer over the cooled sugar cookie crust. Decorate with fruit.
- Cut into slices and serve. Leftovers keep well in the refrigerator for up to 3 days.

Tip: Prepare the cookie "crust" and frosting 1 day in advance-- cover each tightly and keep the cookie at

room temperature and the frosting in the refrigerator.
Frost and assemble the day of serving.

Nutrition Info

Total Fat 14g.
Saturated Fat 5.9g.
Cholesterol 24mg.
Sodium 194mg.
Potassium 158mg.
Total Carbohydrates 44g.
Dietary Fiber 1.4g.

Lunch

Cinnamon Sweet Potatoes With Chicken Sheet Pan

Prep Time 5 mins
Cook Time 1 hr
Total Time 1 hr 5 mins
Servings: 4 servings

Ingredients

- 10 oz. package frozen, sliced carrots
- 10 oz. package frozen, cut sweet potatoes
- 1 lb. frozen chicken breasts (2 breasts)
- 1 tsp. ground cinnamon
- 1/4 tsp. ground cloves

- 1/4 tsp. ground ginger
- 1 tbsp. dried parsley
- oil for cooking

Instructions

- Combine all ingredients in a zipper-top, 1 gallon freezer bag and toss to combine.

- Store in the freezer for up to 4 months.

- When ready to make, preheat oven to 350 F.

- Open the bag and pour in some oil (I used 1/3 cup)

- Close it up again and toss well to coat.

- Pour the contents of the bag out onto a sheet pan with edges.

- Bake for 1 hour or until the chicken reaches at least 165 F. on a meat thermometer.

- Cool slightly and serve.

Nutrition Info

Calories 234 Calories from Fat 27
Total Fat 3g 5%

Cholesterol 72mg 24%
Sodium 237mg 10%
Potassium 984mg 28%
Total Carbohydrates 24g

Dinner

Creamy Fettuccine with Brussels Sprouts & Mushrooms

Cook Time 30 m
Total Time: 30 m
6 servings

Ingredients

- 12 ounces whole-wheat fettuccine
- 1 tablespoon extra-virgin olive oil
- 4 cups sliced mixed mushrooms, such as cremini, oyster and/or shiitake
- 4 cups thinly sliced Brussels sprouts
- 1 tablespoon minced garlic
- ½ cup dry sherry (see Note), or 2 tablespoons sherry vinegar
- 2 cups low-fat milk
- 2 tablespoons all-purpose flour
- ½ teaspoon salt
- ½ teaspoon freshly ground pepper

- 1 cup finely shredded Asiago cheese, plus more for garnish

Instructions

- Cook pasta in a large pot of boiling water until tender, 8 to 10 minutes. Drain, return to the pot and set aside.
- Meanwhile, heat oil in a large skillet over medium heat. Add mushrooms and Brussels sprouts and cook, stirring often, until the mushrooms release their liquid, 8 to 10 minutes.
- Add garlic and cook, stirring, until fragrant, about 1 minute. Add sherry (or vinegar), scraping up any brown bits; bring to a boil and cook, stirring, until almost evaporated, 10 seconds (if using vinegar) or about 1 minute (if using sherry).
- Whisk milk and flour in a bowl; add to the skillet with salt and pepper. Cook, stirring, until the sauce bubbles and thickens, about 2 minutes.
- Stir in Asiago until melted. Add the sauce to the pasta; gently toss. Serve with more cheese, if desired.

Nutrition info

Serving size: about 1? cups

Per serving: 384 calories; 10 g fat(4 g sat); 10 g fiber; 56 g carbohydrates; 18 g protein; 82 mcg folate; 21 mg cholesterol; 8 g sugars; 0 g

Day 18

Breakfast

Broccoli and Cheese Mini Egg Omelets

Total Time:30 minutes
Serving: 4

Ingredients

- 4 cups broccoli florets
- 4 whole large eggs
- 1 cup egg whites
- 1/4 cup reduced fat shredded cheddar (Sargento)
- 1/4 cup good grated cheese like pecorino romano
- 1 tsp olive oil
- salt and fresh pepper
- cooking spray

Instructions

- Preheat oven to 350°.

- Steam broccoli with a little water for about 6-7 minutes.
- When broccoli is cooked, crumble into smaller pieces and add olive oil, salt and pepper. Mix well.
- Spray a standard size non-stick cupcake tin with cooking spray and spoon broccoli mixture evenly into 9 tins.
- In a medium bowl, beat egg whites, eggs, grated cheese, salt and pepper.
- Pour into the greased tins over broccoli until a little more than 3/4 full.
- Top with grated cheddar and bake in the oven until cooked, about 20 minutes. Serve immediately.
- Wrap any leftovers in plastic wrap and store in the refrigerator to enjoy during the week.

Nutrition Info

Calories: 167 calories
Total Fat: 8.5g
Saturated Fat: g
Cholesterol: 170mg

Lunch

The Ultimate Fish Tacos

Prep: 20 min. + marinating Grill: 10 min.
Total Time: 30 min
6 servings

Ingredients

- 1/4 cup olive oil
- 1 teaspoon ground cardamom
- 1 teaspoon paprika
- 1 teaspoon salt
- 1 teaspoon pepper
- 6 mahi mahi fillets (6 ounces each)
- 12 corn tortillas (6 inches)
- 2 cups chopped red cabbage
- 1 cup chopped fresh cilantro
- Salsa verde, optional
- 2 medium limes, cut into wedges
- Hot pepper sauce (Tapatio preferred)

Instructions

- In a 13x9-in. baking dish, whisk the first five ingredients. Add fillets; turn to coat. Refrigerate, covered, 30 minutes.
- Drain fish and discard marinade. On an oiled grill rack, grill mahi mahi, covered, over medium-high heat (or broil 4 in. from heat) until it flakes easily with a fork, 4-5 minutes per

side. Remove fish. Place tortillas on grill rack; heat 30-45 seconds. Keep warm.

- To assemble, divide fish among the tortillas; layer with red cabbage, cilantro and, if desired, salsa verde. Squeeze a little lime juice and hot pepper sauce over fish mixture; fold sides of tortilla over mixture. Serve with lime wedges and additional pepper sauce.

Nutrition Info

2 tacos: 284 calories, 5g fat (1g saturated fat), 124mg cholesterol, 278mg sodium, 26g carbohydrate (2g sugars, 4g fiber), 35g protein

Dinner

Easy Cabbage & White Bean Soup

Total Time: 8hrs 45mins
Serves: 8

Ingredients

- 1 medium yellow onion, coarsely chopped
- 2 medium carrots, coarsely chopped (about 1 cup)
- 1small fennel bulb, cored and coarsely chopped (about 1 cup)

- 3cloves garlic, peeled and crushed
- 2 tablespoons olive oil, plus more for drizzling
- Kosher salt
- 1/4 cup tomato paste
- 6 cups low-sodium vegetable or chicken broth
- 1 very small cabbage (about 1 pound), such as Savoy, cored and thinly shredded
- 2 pieces Parmesan cheese rind (optional)
- 2 (15-ounce) cans cannellini beans, drained but not rinsed
- 1 tablespoon fresh thyme leaves
- 1/4 cup thinly sliced fresh basil leaves
- Freshly ground black pepper
- Red pepper flakes

Instructions

- Place the onion, carrots, fennel, and garlic in the bowl of a food processor fitted with the blade attachment and pulse until very finely chopped but not pureéd. (Alternatively, chop the vegetables as finely as possible with a knife.)

- Heat the oil in a Dutch oven or large soup pot over medium heat until shimmering. Stir in the onion mixture and a big pinch of salt. Cook, stirring occasionally, until very soft, about 10 minutes. The vegetables will nearly melt into a sauce. Increase the heat to medium-high. Stir in the tomato paste and cook, stirring quickly and continuously, until the mixture begins to sizzle, about 1 minute.

- Stir in the broth and bring to a simmer. Stir in the cabbage and another big pinch of salt. Drop in the Parmesan rinds, if using. Simmer until the cabbage is very tender, stirring occaisonally, about 25 minutes. Retrieve the cheese rinds and either discard or nibble on them as a cook's treat.

- Stir in the beans, thyme, and basil and simmer to warm through, about 5 minutes. Taste and season generously with salt, pepper, and pepper flakes as needed. Serve warm, drizzled with olive oil.

Notes

- Shredded cabbage: Instead of a whole cabbage, use 8 cups preshredded cabbage.

- Storage: Leftovers can be stored in an airtight container in the refrigerator for up to 5 days or frozen for up to 2 months.

Nutrition Info

Calories 253

Fat 6.1 g
Saturated 1.2 g
Carbs 37.6 g
Fiber 7.9 g
Sugars 7.2 g
Protein

Day 19

Breakfast

The Best Avocado Toast

Prep Time: 20 minutes
Total Time: 20 minutes
Serving: 4 slices

Ingredients

- 4 slices thick whole grain bread (or gluten-free equivalent)
- 1 large ripe avocado
- 1/3 cup frozen shelled edamame
- 1 lime
- 1 scallion (sliced thinly)
- 1/2 cup raw fresh corn kernels (1 ear)
- 1/2 cup tomato (diced)
- 1/2 cup cilantro (chopped)
- 1/4 cup hemp seeds (optional)

- salt to taste
- crushed red pepper flakes (to taste)
- olive oil (for drizzling)

Instructions

- Toast the bread.
- Soak the edamame in warm water in a small bowl.
- Cut the corn off the cob and measure out 1/2 cup (save remaining corn for another use).
- Mash the edamame in a small bowl and then mash in the avocado.
- Add the sliced scallions and corn to the avocado/edamame mixture.
- Add the juice from half of the lime along with a sprinkle of salt, mix, and taste. Add more lime juice or salt as needed.
- When the toast is done, rub a cut garlic clove over the surface of each piece of toast.
- Spread the avocado mixture evenly onto each piece of toast.
- Top each slice with a drizzle of olive oil, crushed red pepper flakes, hemp seeds, tomato, and cilantro. You can also add a sprinkle of salt and lime juice if you like.

Nutrition Info

Calories 280

Total Fat 16.8g
Cholesterol 0mg
Sodium 738.1mg
Total Carbohydrate 26.8g

Lunch

Cucumber Sandwiches

Prep Time 15 minutes
Total Time 15 minutes
Servings 30 tea sandwiches

Ingredients

- 8 oz cream cheese softened
- 3 tablespoons mayonnaise
- 2 teaspoons chopped fresh dill
- 1 teaspoon chopped fresh chives
- 1/4 teaspoon garlic powder
- salt & pepper to taste
- 1 long English cucumber thinly sliced
- 1 loaf sliced bread crusts removed

Instructions

- With a hand mixer mix cream cheese and mayonnaise in a small bowl until smooth. Stir in herbs, garlic powder and salt and pepper to taste.

- Spread bread slices with cream cheese mixture.

- Thinly slice cucumbers. Layer over half of the bread slices. Top with additional herbs if desired.

- Top with remaining bread slice, remove crusts if desired and cut each sandwich into 3 pieces.
- Serve immediately or cover and store up to 24 hours.

Nutrition Info

Calories: 39
Fat: 3g
Saturated Fat: 1g
Cholesterol: 8mg
Sodium: 37mg
Potassium: 25mg

Dinner

Stuffed Sweet Potato with Hummus Dressing

Prep 15 m
Cook Time: 5m

Total Time 20 m
1 serving

Ingredients

- 1 large sweet potato, scrubbed
- ¾ cup chopped kale
- 1 cup canned black beans, rinsed
- ¼ cup hummus
- 2 tablespoons water

Instructions

- Prick sweet potato all over with a fork. Microwave on High until cooked through, 7 to 10 minutes. Meanwhile, wash kale and drain, allowing water to cling to the leaves. Place in a medium saucepan; cover and cook over medium-high heat, stirring once or twice, until wilted. Add beans; add a tablespoon or two of water if the pot is dry.
- Continue cooking, uncovered, stirring occasionally, until the mixture is steaming hot, 1 to 2 minutes. Split the sweet potato open and top with the kale and bean mixture.
- Combine hummus and 2 tablespoons water in a small dish. Add additional water as needed to reach desired consistency.
- Drizzle the hummus dressing over the stuffed sweet potato.

Nutrition info

472 calories
7 g fat(1 g sat)
22 g fiber
85 g carbohydrates
21 g protein

Day 20

Breakfast

Sausage and Mushroom Strata

Total Time:9 hours
Prep Time:10 minutes + overnight to set (or 8 hours)
Cook Time:50 minutes
8 servings

Ingredients

- 8 oz wheat ciabatta bread, cut into 1-inch cubes (Chabaso)
- 12 oz turkey breakfast sausage (I used Jenny-O in frozen section)
- 2 cups fat-free milk
- 1-1/2 cup (4 ounces) reduced-fat shredded sharp cheddar cheese

- 3 large eggs
- 12 oz egg substitute, like egg beaters
- 1/2 cup chopped green onions
- 1 cup sliced mushrooms
- 1/2 tsp paprika
- salt and fresh pepper
- 2 tbsp grated parmesan cheese

Instructions

- Preheat oven to 400°.
- Arrange bread cubes on a baking sheet.
- Bake at 400° for 8 minutes or until toasted.
- Heat a medium skillet over medium-high heat.
- Add sausage to pan; cook 7 minutes or until browned, stirring to crumble.
- Combine milk, cheese, eggs, egg substitute, parmesan cheese, paprika, salt and pepper in a large bowl, stirring with a whisk.
- Add bread, sausage, scallions and mushrooms, tossing well to coat bread.
- Spoon mixture into a 13×9-inch baking dish.
- Cover and refrigerate 8 hours or overnight.
- Preheat oven to 350°.
- Uncover casserole.
- Bake at 350° for 50 minutes or until set and lightly browned.
- Cut into 8 pieces; serve immediately.

Nutrition Info

Calories: 288.2 calories
Total Fat: 12.4g
Saturated Fat: 1.8g

Lunch

Grilled tofu burgers with mushrooms & blue cheese

Prep Time: 5 minutes
Cook Time: 10 minutes
Serving: 4 burgers

Ingredients

- 2 blocks of super firm tofu, drained and pressed (if necessary)
- 2 tablespoons olive oil
- 1 tablespoon Barbecue Spice Rub
- 1 tablespoon butter
- 8 ounces button mushrooms, sliced
- 1 medium onion, sliced
- 4 hamburger buns
- 4 ounces blue cheese
- Barbecue sauce

Instructions

- Preheat the grill over high heat. While the grill is heating, slice the tofu into burger-sized planks, brush with olive oil and sprinkle with spice rub. Set aside.
- In a medium skillet over high heat, melt the butter. Add in the mushrooms and onions and continue to cook over high heat until the veggies are soft and beginning to brown. Set aside.
- When the grill is heated up, place the tofu on the grill grates, close lid and sear for 2-3 minutes, or until the tofu is browned. Flip and repeat on the other side. If you're using good firm tofu, you don't need to "cook" it as much as just warm it up and sear it. Remove from the grill.
- To assemble the burgers, stack a tofu slice on the bottom of a bun, top with 1/4 of the mushroom mixture, 1/4 of the blue cheese and a big dollop of barbecue sauce. Place top of bun on and serve with plenty of napkins.

Nutrition Info

Calories: 401 cal

Dinner

Creamy Lentils with Kale Artichoke Saute

Prep/Total Time: 30 min

Serving 4 serves

Ingredients

- 1/2 cup dried red lentils, rinsed and sorted
- 1/4 teaspoon dried oregano
- 1/8 teaspoon pepper
- 1-1/4 cups vegetable broth
- 1/4 teaspoon sea salt, divided
- 1 tablespoon olive oil or grapeseed oil
- 16 cups chopped fresh kale (about 12 ounces)
- 1 can (14 ounces) water-packed artichoke hearts, drained and chopped
- 3 garlic cloves, minced
- 1/2 teaspoon Italian seasoning
- 2 tablespoons grated Romano cheese
- 2 cups hot cooked brown or basmati rice

Instructions

- Place first four ingredients and 1/8 teaspoon salt in a small saucepan; bring to a boil. Reduce heat; simmer, covered, until lentils are tender and liquid is almost absorbed, 12-15 minutes. Remove from heat.
- In a 6-qt. stockpot, heat oil over medium heat. Add kale and remaining salt; cook, covered, until kale is wilted, 4-5 minutes, stirring

occasionally. Add artichoke hearts, garlic and Italian seasoning; cook and stir 3 minutes. Remove from heat; stir in cheese.

- Serve lentils and kale mixture over rice.

Nutrition Info

321 calories, 6g fat (2g saturated fat), 1mg cholesterol, 661mg sodium, 53g carbohydrate (1g sugars, 5g fiber), 15g protein.

Day 21

Breakfast

Eggs and Tomato Breakfast Melts

Total Time:10 minutes
Prep Time:3 minutes
Cook Time:7 minutes
4 servings

Ingredients

- 2 whole grain English muffins, split
- 1 teaspoon olive oil
- 8 egg whites, whisked
- 4 scallions, finely chopped
- kosher salt, to taste

- black pepper, to taste
- 2 oz (about 1/2 cup) reduced-fat Mexican cheese blend, grated
- 1/2 cup grape or cherry heirloom tomatoes, quartered

Instructions

- Preheat the broiler on high.
- Place muffins, cut side up, on a baking sheet and broil for 2 minutes or until beginning to lightly brown on edges. (Or you can do this in your toaster oven)
- Heat a medium skillet on medium heat.
- Add oil and sauté 3 of the scallions about 2 to 3 minutes.
- Add the egg whites, season with salt and pepper and cook, mixing with a wooden spoon until cooked through.
- Divide on toasted muffins and top with tomatoes, cheese and remaining scallions.
- Broil for 1 to 1 1/2 minutes or until cheese has melted, careful not to burn.

Nutrition Info

Calories: 160 calories
Total Fat: 5g
Saturated Fat: 0.5g
Cholesterol: 8mg

Lunch

Zucchini Noodles Pad Thai

Prep: 45 m
Cook: 12 m
Total Time: 57 m

Ingredients

- 3 large zucchini
- 1/4 cup chicken stock
- 2 1/2 tablespoons tamarind paste
- 2 tablespoons low-sodium soy sauce
- 2 tablespoons oyster sauce
- 1 1/2 tablespoons Asian chile pepper sauce
- 1 tablespoon Worcestershire sauce
- 1 tablespoon fresh lime juice
- 1 tablespoon white sugar
- 2 tablespoons sesame oil
- 1 tablespoon chopped garlic
- 12 ounces skinless, boneless chicken breasts, cut into 1-inch cubes
- 8 ounces peeled and deveined shrimp
- 2 eggs, beaten
- 2 tablespoons water, or as needed (optional)
- 3 cups bean sprouts, divided
- 6 green onions, chopped into 1-inch pieces

- 2 tablespoons chopped unsalted dry-roasted peanuts
- 1/4 cup chopped fresh basil

Instructions

Make zucchini noodles using a spiralizer.
- Whisk chicken stock, tamarind paste, soy sauce, oyster sauce, chile pepper sauce, Worcestershire sauce, lime juice, and sugar together in a small bowl to make a smooth sauce.
- Heat sesame oil in a wok or large skillet over high heat. Add garlic and stir until fragrant, about 10 seconds. Add chicken and shrimp; cook and stir until chicken is no longer pink in the center and the juices run clear, 5 to 7 minutes.
- Push chicken and shrimp to the sides of the wok to make a space in the center. Pour eggs and scramble until firm, 2 to 3 minutes. Add zucchini noodles and sauce; cook and stir, adding water if needed, about 3 minutes. Add 2 cups bean sprouts and green onions; cook and stir until combined, 1 to 2 minutes.
- Remove wok from heat and sprinkle peanuts over noodles. Serve garnished with remaining 1 cup bean sprouts and fresh basil.

370 calories
14.5 g fat
28.1 g carbohydrates
35.6 g protein
222 mg cholesterol
671 mg sodium

Dinner

Asparagus Turkey Stir-Fry

Prep/Total Time: 20 min.
4 servings

Ingredients

- 2 teaspoons cornstarch
- 1/4 cup chicken broth
- 1 tablespoon lemon juice
- 1 teaspoon soy sauce
- 1 pound turkey breast tenderloins, cut into 1/2-inch strips
- 1 garlic clove, minced
- 2 tablespoons canola oil, divided
- 1 pound fresh asparagus, trimmed and cut into 1-1/2-inch pieces
- 1 jar (2 ounces) sliced pimientos, drained

Instructions

- In a small bowl, combine the cornstarch, broth, lemon juice and soy sauce until smooth; set aside. In a large skillet or wok, stir-fry turkey and garlic in 1 tablespoon oil until meat is no longer pink; remove and keep warm.
- Stir-fry asparagus in remaining oil until crisp-tender. Add pimientos. Stir broth mixture and add to the pan; cook and stir for 1 minute or until thickened. Return turkey to the pan; heat through.

Nutrition Info

205 calories
9g fat (1g saturated fat)
56mg cholesterol
204mg sodium
5g carbohydrate (1g sugars, 1g fiber)
28g protein

Day 22

Breakfast

Fruit-N-Grain Breakfast Salad

Total Time:20 minutes
Prep Time:5 minutes
Cook Time:15 minutes
8 servings

Ingredients

- 3 cups water
- 1/4 teaspoon salt
- 3/4 cup quick-cooking brown rice
- 3/4 cup bulgur
- 1 Granny Smith apple
- 1 Red Delicious apple
- 1 orange
- 1 cup raisins
- 1 container (8-ounce) low fat vanilla yogurt

Instructions

- In large pot, heat water and salt to boiling over high heat. Add rice and bulgur; reduce heat to low, cover, and cook 10 minutes. Remove from heat and set aside, covered 2 minutes. Spread hot grains on baking sheet to cool (this will make them fluffier). Grains can be prepared the night before and kept refrigerated.

- Just before serving, prepare fruit: Core and chop apples; peel orange and cut into sections.

Add apples, orange, and raisins to grain mixture. Stir in yogurt to coat grains and fruit.

Nutrition Info

Calories: 187
Protein: 4g
Fat: 1g
Carbohydrates: 40g
Fiber: 5g
Sodium: 117mg
Cholesterol: 1mg

Lunch

15 Minute Healthy Roasted Chicken and Veggies (One Pan)

Prep Time 5 minutes
Cook Time 15 minutes
Total Time 20 minutes
Servings 2

Ingredients

- 2 medium chicken breasts chopped
- 1 cup bell pepper chopped (any colors you like)
- 1/2 onion chopped
- 1 zucchini chopped

- 1 cup broccoli florets
- 1/2 cup tomatoes chopped or plum/grape
- 2 tablespoons olive oil
- 1/2 teaspoon salt
- 1/2 teaspoon black pepper
- 1 teaspoon italian seasoning
- 1/4 teaspoon paprika optional

Instructions

- Preheat oven to 500 degree F.
- Chop all the veggies into large pieces. In another cutting board chop the chicken into cubes. Place the chicken and veggies in a medium roasting dish or sheet pan. Add the olive oil, salt and pepper, italian seasoning, and paprika. Toss to combine.
- Bake for 15 minutes or until the veggies are charred and chicken is cooked. Enjoy with rice, pasta, or a salad.

Nutrition Info

Calories 242
Total Fat 15.2g 23%
Cholesterol 55.7mg 19%
Sodium 357mg 15%

Dinner

Sweet Onion & Sausage Spaghetti

Prep/Total Time: 30 min.
4 servings

Ingredients

- 6 ounces uncooked whole wheat spaghetti
- 3/4 pound Italian turkey sausage links, casings removed
- 2 teaspoons olive oil
- 1 sweet onion, thinly sliced
- 1 pint cherry tomatoes, halved
- 1/2 cup loosely packed fresh basil leaves, thinly sliced
- 1/2 cup half-and-half cream
- Shaved Parmesan cheese, optional

Instructions

- Cook spaghetti according to package Instructions. Meanwhile, in a large nonstick skillet over medium heat, cook sausage in oil for 5 minutes. Add onion; cook 8-10 minutes longer or until meat is no longer pink and onion is tender.
- Stir in tomatoes and basil; heat through. Add cream; bring to a boil. Drain spaghetti; toss

with sausage mixture. Garnish with cheese if desired.

Nutrition Info

334 calories
12g fat (4g saturated fat)
46mg cholesterol
378mg sodium
41g carbohydrate
17g protein.

Day 23

Breakfast

Spinach, Mushroom, and Feta Cheese Scramble

Prep/Total Time: 15 min.
1 Servings

Ingredients

- Cooking spray
- ½ cup fresh mushrooms, sliced
- 1 cup fresh spinach, chopped
- 1 whole egg and 2 egg whites
- 2 tablespoons feta cheese
- Pepper to taste

Instructions

- Heat an 8-inch non-stick sauté pan over medium heat. Spray with cooking spray and add mushrooms and spinach.

- Sauté mushrooms and spinach for 2-3 minutes or until the spinach has wilted.

- Whisk the egg and egg whites in a bowl with feta cheese and pepper if desired. Pour egg mixture over vegetables in the pan.

- Continue to cook eggs while stirring with a spatula for another 3-4 minutes or until the eggs are cooked through.

Nutrition Info

Calories 236.5
Total Fat 11.4 g
Saturated Fat 5.9 g

Lunch

Roasted Vegetable and Farro Salad

Prep Time: 20 minutes

Total Time: 20 minutes

Servings: 3

Ingredients

Farro:

- 1 1/2 - 2 cups semi-pearled farro

Vegetables:

- 2 Zucchini summer squash, cut into 3-4 inch long quarters
- 2 large Portobello mushrooms stem and spines removes and sliced
- 3 large Bell peppers core and seeds removed and cut into wide, 3-4 inch long slices
- 1 large Red onion cut into chunks
- Olive oil
- Salt and pepper

Dressing:

- 2 Tbsp Balsamic vinegar
- 1/2 cup Olive oil
- 1/2 tsp Dijon mustard
- Leaves from 1 sprig of fresh thyme
- Salt
- Pepper

To serve:

- 1 cup crumbled feta cheese
- Additional fresh thyme leaves

Instructions

- Cook the farro: Bring a large pot of water to a boil over high heat. Add farro and boil until al dente, about 20 minutes. Drain and remove to a bowl. If making ahead, allow to cool at room temperature for 10-15 minutes, then cover and refrigerate. Otherwise, set aside while you roast the vegetables.
- Roast the vegetables: Preheat the oven to 450F. Place all the vegetables in a large bowl. Drizzle with a bit of olive oil and season with salt and pepper. Scatter evenly over a large baking sheet. Roast 30 minutes in the preheated oven, stirring once. Remove from oven and switch oven to broil with oven rack about 6-8 inches from the heat. Broil for 3-5 minutes or until lightly charred. Remove from oven and let cool 5 minutes them remove to a large bowl.
- Prepare the dressing: Whisk all the dressing ingredients together in a small bowl. Set aside.
- *If you made the farro ahead, remove from fridge to come to room temperature or re-warm slightly to serve.

To serve

- Toss the farro with 1 Tbsp (or so) of the dressing. Season with a bit of salt and pepper, then scatter a large spoonful onto each of the serving plates. Drizzle the roasted vegetables with some of the dressing, until evenly moistened. Add the crumbled feta and stir to combine. Spoon vegetables/feta over farro on serving plates. Garnish with a few more thyme leaves and some freshly ground pepper. Serve with any additional dressing, for drizzling as needed.

Nutrition Info

Calories: 482 kcal

Dinner

White Beans & Bow Ties

Prep/Total Time: 25 min.
Makes 4 servings

Ingredients

- 2-1/2 cups uncooked whole wheat bow tie pasta (about 6 ounces)

- 1 tablespoon olive oil
- 1 medium zucchini, sliced
- 2 garlic cloves, minced
- 2 large tomatoes, chopped (about 2-1/2 cups)
- 1 can (15 ounces) cannellini beans, rinsed and drained
- 1 can (2-1/4 ounces) sliced ripe olives, drained
- 3/4 teaspoon freshly ground pepper
- 1/2 cup crumbled feta cheese

Instructions

- Cook pasta according to package Instructions. Drain, reserving 1/2 cup pasta water.
- Meanwhile, in a large skillet, heat oil over medium-high heat; saute zucchini until crisp-tender, 2-4 minutes. Add garlic; cook and stir 30 seconds. Stir in tomatoes, beans, olives and pepper; bring to a boil. Reduce heat; simmer, uncovered, until tomatoes are softened, 3-5 minutes, stirring occasionally.
- Stir in pasta and enough pasta water to moisten as desired. Stir in cheese.

Tip: Boost protein in meatless pasta dishes by using whole wheat noodles, adding white beans or stirring in a little cheese—or all three!

Nutrition Info

1-1/2 cups: 348 calories, 9g fat (2g saturated fat), 8mg cholesterol, 394mg sodium, 52g carbohydrate (4g sugars, 11g fiber), 15g protein.

Day 24

Breakfast

Overnight Oats

Prep Time: 5 minutes
Cook Time: 0 minutes
Total Time: 5 minutes
1 serving

Ingredients

- 1/2 cup homemade muesli, or old-fashioned oats plus ¼ teaspoon ground cinnamon
- 1 tablespoon chia seeds
- 1 tablespoon almond butter or peanut butter
- ½ cup milk of choice for a very thick consistency
- ½ cup fruit (I like fresh or frozen blueberries or raspberries, or sliced fresh strawberries)
- Drizzle of maple syrup or honey, if desired

Instructions

- In a jar or bowl (a 14-ounce working jar or 1-pint mason jar is perfect), combine the muesli (or old-fashioned oats and cinnamon), chia seeds and nut butter. Add a splash of the milk and mix the nut butter into the oats. Then add the rest of the milk and stir to combine.
- Top with your fruit of choice. (If you used more milk than ½ cup and you want your fruit to stay on top, wait to top the oats until you're ready to serve. If you're using fruit that doesn't store well, like sliced apple or banana, wait to top the oats until you're ready to serve.)
- Place the lid on the jar and refrigerate overnight, or up to 5 days. When you're ready to serve, add a drizzle of maple syrup or honey if you'd like, and enjoy chilled.

Nutrition Info

Calories: 243 calories
Total Fat: 11g
Saturated Fat: g
Cholesterol: mg
Sodium: 95mg

Lunch

Chickpea Mint Tabbouleh

Prep/Total Time: 30 min.
4 servings

Ingredients

- 1 cup bulgur
- 2 cups water
- 1 cup fresh or frozen peas (about 5 ounces), thawed
- 1 can (15 ounces) chickpeas or garbanzo beans, rinsed and drained
- 1/2 cup minced fresh parsley
- 1/4 cup minced fresh mint
- 1/4 cup olive oil
- 2 tablespoons julienned soft sun-dried tomatoes (not packed in oil)
- 2 tablespoons lemon juice
- 1/2 teaspoon salt
- 1/4 teaspoon pepper

Instructions

- In a large saucepan, combine bulgur and water; bring to a boil. Reduce heat; simmer, covered, 10 minutes. Stir in fresh or frozen peas; cook, covered, until bulgur and peas are tender, about 5 minutes.
- Transfer to a large bowl. Stir in remaining ingredients. Serve warm or refrigerate and serve cold.

Nutrition Info

1 cup: 380 calories
16g fat (2g saturated fat)
0 cholesterol
450mg sodium
51g carbohydrate (6g sugars, 11g fiber)
11g protein.

Dinner

Black Bean & Sweet Potato Rice Bowls

Prep/Total Time: 30 min.
4 servings

Ingredients

- 3/4 cup uncooked long grain rice
- 1/4 teaspoon garlic salt
- 1-1/2 cups water
- 3 tablespoons olive oil, divided
- 1 large sweet potato, peeled and diced
- 1 medium red onion, finely chopped
- 4 cups chopped fresh kale (tough stems removed)
- 1 can (15 ounces) black beans, rinsed and drained

- 2 tablespoons sweet chili sauce
- Lime wedges, optional
- Additional sweet chili sauce, optional

Instructions

- Place rice, garlic salt and water in a large saucepan; bring to a boil. Reduce heat; simmer, covered, until water is absorbed and rice is tender, 15-20 minutes. Remove from heat; let stand 5 minutes.
- Meanwhile, in a large skillet, heat 2 tablespoons oil over medium-high heat; saute sweet potato 8 minutes. Add onion; cook and stir until potato is tender, 4-6 minutes. Add kale; cook and stir until tender, 3-5 minutes. Stir in beans; heat through.
- Gently stir 2 tablespoons chili sauce and remaining oil into rice; add to potato mixture. If desired, serve with lime wedges and additional chili sauce.

Nutrition Info

2 cups: 435 calories, 11g fat (2g saturated fat), 0 cholesterol, 405mg sodium, 74g carbohydrate (15g sugars, 8g fiber), 10g protein.

Day 25

Breakfast

The Perfect Granola

Total Time: 20mins
Serves: 10

Ingredients

- 4 cups oats
- 3 cups of chopped nuts (mixture of whatever you like)
- 2 cups raisins (or other sweet dried fruit)
- 1 cup sunflower seeds (whatever) or 1 cup pumpkin seeds (whatever)
- 1/2 cup honey
- 1/2 cup extra light olive oil (or another neutral tasting oil)
- 1/4 cup maple syrup

Instructions

- Mix it all together.
- Spread on baking sheet.
- Bake at 325 for 13 minutes stirring once.

Nutrition Info

Serving Size: 1 (182 g)

Servings Per Recipe: 10
Calories 823.7
Calories from Fat 391 48%
Total Fat 43.5 g 66%
Saturated Fat 5.8 g 29%
Cholesterol 0 mg

Lunch

Grilled Veggie Sandwich

Prep: 30 m
Cook: 20 m
Total Time: 50 m
4 servings

Ingredients

- 1/4 cup mayonnaise
- 3 cloves garlic, minced
- 1 tablespoon lemon juice
- 1/8 cup olive oil
- 1 cup sliced red bell peppers
- 1 small zucchini, sliced
- 1 red onion, sliced
- 1 small yellow squash, sliced
- 2 (4-x6-inch) focaccia bread pieces, split horizontally
- 1/2 cup crumbled feta cheese

Instructions

- In a bowl, mix the mayonnaise, minced garlic, and lemon juice. Set aside in the refrigerator.
- Preheat the grill for high heat.
- Brush vegetables with olive oil on each side. Brush grate with oil. Place bell peppers and zucchini closest to the middle of the grill, and set onion and squash pieces around them. Cook for about 3 minutes, turn, and cook for another 3 minutes. The peppers may take a bit longer. Remove from grill, and set aside.
- Spread some of the mayonnaise mixture on the cut sides of the bread, and sprinkle each one with feta cheese. Place on the grill cheese side up, and cover with lid for 2 to 3 minutes. This will warm the bread, and slightly melt the cheese. Watch carefully so the bottoms don't burn. Remove from grill, and layer with the vegetables. Enjoy as open faced grilled sandwiches.

Nutrition Info

393 calories
23.8 g fat
36.5 g carbohydrates
9.2 g protein
22 mg cholesterol

623 mg sodium.

Dinner

Spinach-Orzo Salad with Chickpeas

Prep/Total Time: 25 min.
12 servings (3/4 cup each)

Ingredients

- 1 can (14-1/2 ounces) reduced-sodium chicken broth
- 1-1/2 cups uncooked whole wheat orzo pasta
- 4 cups fresh baby spinach
- 2 cups grape tomatoes, halved
- 2 cans (15 ounces each) chickpeas or garbanzo beans, rinsed and drained
- 3/4 cup chopped fresh parsley
- 2 green onions, chopped
- DRESSING:
- 1/4 cup olive oil
- 3 tablespoons lemon juice
- 3/4 teaspoon salt
- 1/4 teaspoon garlic powder
- 1/4 teaspoon hot pepper sauce
- 1/4 teaspoon pepper

Instructions

- In a large saucepan, bring broth to a boil. Stir in orzo; return to a boil. Reduce heat; simmer, covered, until al dente, 8-10 minutes.
- In a large bowl, toss spinach and warm orzo, allowing spinach to wilt slightly. Add tomatoes, chickpeas, parsley and green onions.
- Whisk together dressing ingredients. Toss with salad.

Nutrition Info

122 calories
5g fat (1g saturated fat)
0 cholesterol
259mg sodium
16g carbohydrate (1g sugars, 4g fiber)
4g protein

Day 26

Breakfast

Steel Cut Oat Blueberry Pancakes

Prep Time 5 Minutes
Cook Time 10 Minutes
Total Time
Servings 10 People

Ingredients

- 1-1/2 cups Water
- 1/2 cup Steel Cut Oats or Organic Steel Cut Oats
- 1/8 tsp Sea Salt
- 1 cup Whole Wheat Pastry Flour or Organic Whole Wheat Pastry Flour
- 1/2 tsp Baking Powder
- 1/2 tsp Baking Soda
- 1 Egg
- 1 cup Milk
- 1/2 cup Greek Yogurt vanilla flavor
- 1 cup Frozen Blueberries
- 1/2 cup Agave Nectar +2 tbsp

Instructions

- In a medium pot bring water to a boil and add steel cut oats and salt. Reduce heat to a low simmer and cook until oats are tender, about 10 minutes. Remove from heat and set aside.
- In a medium mixing bowl combine whole wheat pastry flour, baking powder and soda, egg, milk and yogurt. Mix until a batter is formed. Gently fold in blueberries and cooked oats.
- Using a griddle or non-stick skillet heated over medium and coated with cooking spray spoon one quarter cup of batter onto surface and

cook until they begin to bubble and are slightly golden, about 2 - 3 minutes per side, working in batches if needed.

- Garnish each pancake with about one tablespooon agave nectar.

Nutrition Info

Calories257 cal
Fat7 g
Carbs46 g
Protein14 g

Lunch

Roasted Sweet Potato & Chickpea Pitas

Prep/Total Time: 30 min.
6 servings

Ingredients

- 2 medium sweet potatoes (about 1-1/4 pounds), peeled and cubed
- 2 cans (15 ounces each) chickpeas or garbanzo beans, rinsed and drained
- 1 medium red onion, chopped
- 3 tablespoons canola oil, divided
- 2 teaspoons garam masala

- 1/2 teaspoon salt, divided
- 2 garlic cloves, minced
- 1 cup plain Greek yogurt
- 1 tablespoon lemon juice
- 1 teaspoon ground cumin
- 2 cups arugula or baby spinach
- 12 whole wheat pita pocket halves, warmed
- 1/4 cup minced fresh cilantro

Instructions

- Preheat oven to 400°. Place potatoes in a large microwave-safe bowl; microwave, covered, on high 5 minutes. Stir in chickpeas and onion; toss with 2 tablespoons oil, garam masala and 1/4 teaspoon salt.
- Spread into a 15x10x1-in. pan. Roast until potatoes are tender, about 15 minutes. Cool slightly.
- Place garlic and remaining oil in a small microwave-safe bowl; microwave on high until garlic is lightly browned, 1 to 1-1/2 minutes. Stir in yogurt, lemon juice, cumin and remaining salt.
- Toss potato mixture with arugula. Spoon into pitas; top with sauce and cilantro.

Nutrition Info

2 filled pita halves: 462 calories

15g fat (3g saturated fat)
10mg cholesterol, 662mg sodium
72g carbohydrate (13g sugars, 12g fiber)
14g protein.

Dinner

Cilantro Lime Shrimp Recipe

Prep Time 10 minutes
Cook Time 5 minutes
Total Time 15 minutes
Servings 4

Ingredients

- 1 lb tail-on jumbo shrimp peeled and deveined
- 1/4 teaspoon salt or to taste
- Big pinch of cayenne pepper
- 2 tablespoons olive oil
- 4 cloves garlic minced
- 3 tablespoons chopped cilantro stems and leaves
- 1 tablespoon unsalted butter
- 2 tablespoons lime juice
- Fresh lemon wedges

Instructions

- Season the shrimp with salt and cayenne pepper.
- Heat up a cast-iron skillet, add the olive oil, garlic and lightly saute before adding the shrimp.
  - Stir and cook until the shrimp is half cooked.
  - Add the cilantro, butter, stir to combine well with the shrimp.
  - Add the lime juice and continue to cook the shrimp. Turn off the heat when the lime juice dries up and the shrimp is nicely cooked and slightly charred on the surface.
  - Serve immediately with some fresh lime wedges.

Nutrition Info

Calories 171 Calories from Fat 89
Total Fat 9.9g 15%
Saturated Fat 2.8g 14%
Cholesterol 241mg 80%
Sodium 1485mg

Day 27

Breakfast

Red Velvet Pancakes with Cream Cheese Topping

Prep 20 min
Total 20 min
Servings 14

Ingredients

- 4 oz (half of 8-oz package) cream cheese, softened
- 1/4 cup butter, softened
- 3 tablespoons milk
- 2 cups powdered sugar Pancakes
- 2 cups Original Bisquick™ mix
- 1 tablespoon granulated sugar
- 1 tablespoon unsweetened baking cocoa
- 1 cup milk
- 1 to 1 1/2 teaspoons red paste food color*
- 2 eggs

Instructions

- In medium bowl, beat cream cheese, butter and 3 tablespoons milk with electric mixer on low speed until smooth. Gradually beat in 2 cups powdered sugar, 1 cup at a time, on low speed until topping is smooth. Cover; set aside.
- In large bowl, stir all pancake ingredients except powdered sugar with wire whisk until well blended. Heat griddle or skillet over medium-high heat (375°F). (To test griddle, sprinkle with a few drops of water. If bubbles

jump around, heat is just right.) Brush with vegetable oil if necessary or spray with cooking spray before heating.

- For each pancake, pour slightly less than 1/4 cup batter onto hot griddle. Cook 2 to 3 minutes or until bubbles form on top and edges are dry. Turn; cook other side until golden brown.
- Spoon cream cheese topping into resealable food-storage plastic bag; seal bag. Cut off tiny corner of bag; squeeze bag to drizzle topping over pancakes. Sprinkle with powdered sugar.

Nutrition Info

Serving Size: 1 Serving
Calories 450
Calories from Fat 170

Lunch

Lime Chicken Tacos

Prep: 10 min.
Cook: 5-1/2 hours
Makes 6 servings

Ingredients

- 1-1/2 pounds boneless skinless chicken breast halves
- 3 tablespoons lime juice
- 1 tablespoon chili powder
- 1 cup frozen corn, thawed
- 1 cup chunky salsa
- 12 fat-free flour tortillas (6 inches), warmed
- Sour cream, pickled onions, shredded lettuce and shredded cheddar or cotija cheese, optional

Instructions

- Place chicken in a 3-qt. slow cooker. Combine lime juice and chili powder; pour over chicken. Cook, covered, on low until chicken is tender, 5-6 hours.
- Remove chicken. When cool enough to handle, shred meat with two forks; return to slow cooker. Stir in corn and salsa. Cook, covered, on low until heated through, about 30 minutes. Place filling on tortillas; if desired, serve with sour cream, pickled onions, lettuce and cheese.

Nutrition Info

2 tacos:
291 calories
3g fat (1g saturated fat)
63mg cholesterol
674mg sodium

37g carbohydrate (2g sugars, 2g fiber)
28g protein.

Dinner

Chicken & Goat Cheese Skillet

Prep/Total Time: 20 min.
2 servings

Ingredients

- 1/2 pound boneless skinless chicken breasts, cut into 1-inch pieces
- 1/4 teaspoon salt
- 1/8 teaspoon pepper
- 2 teaspoons olive oil
- 1 cup cut fresh asparagus (1-inch pieces)
- 1 garlic clove, minced
- 3 plum tomatoes, chopped
- 3 tablespoons 2% milk
- 2 tablespoons herbed fresh goat cheese, crumbled
- Hot cooked rice or pasta
- Additional goat cheese, optional

Instructions

- Toss chicken with salt and pepper. In a large skillet, heat oil over medium-high heat; saute chicken until no longer pink, 4-6 minutes. Remove from pan; keep warm.
- Add asparagus to skillet; cook and stir over medium-high heat 1 minute. Add garlic; cook and stir 30 seconds. Stir in tomatoes, milk and 2 tablespoons cheese; cook, covered, over medium heat until cheese begins to melt, 2-3 minutes. Stir in chicken. Serve with rice. If desired, top with additional cheese.

Nutrition Info

1-1/2 cups chicken mixture: 251 calories, 11g fat (3g saturated fat), 74mg cholesterol, 447mg sodium, 8g

Day 28

Breakfast

Very Berry Muesli ('mew-slee')

Prep time:5 MIN
Servings: 5 Servings

Ingredients:

- 1 cup low fat fruit yogurt

- 1 cup old-fashioned rolled oats (raw)
- 1/2 cup non-fat or 1% milk
- 1/2 cup dried fruit (try raisins, apricots, dates)
- 1/2 cup chopped apple
- 1/2 cup frozen blueberries
- 1/4 cup chopped, toasted walnuts

Instructions

- In medium bowl, mix oats, yogurt, and milk.
- Cover and refrigerate for 6 to 12 hours.
- Add dried and fresh fruit, and mix gently.
- Serve scoops of muesli in small dishes. Sprinkle each serving with chopped nuts.
- Refrigerate leftovers within 2 hours.

Nutrition Info

Total Fat 4.2g.
Saturated Fat 2.6g.
Sodium 28mg.
Total Carbohydrates 18g.
Dietary Fiber 2.1g.
Protein 1.8g.

Lunch

Strawberry-Blue Cheese Steak Salad

Prep/Total Time: 30 min.
4 servings

Ingredients

- 1 beef top sirloin steak (3/4 inch thick and 1 pound)
- 1/2 teaspoon salt
- 1/4 teaspoon pepper
- 2 teaspoons olive oil
- 2 tablespoons lime juice
- SALAD:
- 1 bunch romaine, torn (about 10 cups)
- 2 cups fresh strawberries, halved
- 1/4 cup thinly sliced red onion
- 1/4 cup crumbled blue cheese
- 1/4 cup chopped walnuts, toasted
- Reduced-fat balsamic vinaigrette

Instructions

- Season steak with salt and pepper. In a large skillet, heat oil over medium heat. Add steak; cook 5-7 minutes on each side until meat reaches desired doneness (for medium-rare, a thermometer should read 135°; medium, 140°; medium-well, 145°). Remove from pan; let stand 5 minutes. Cut steak into bite-size strips; toss with lime juice.

- On a platter, combine romaine, strawberries and onion; top with steak. Sprinkle with cheese and walnuts. Serve with vinaigrette.

Nutrition Info

1 serving: 289 calories
15g fat (4g saturated fat)
52mg cholesterol
452mg sodium
12g carbohydrate (5g sugars, 4g fiber)
29g protein.

Dinner

Weeknight Chicken Chop Suey

Prep/Total Time: 30 min.
6 servings

Ingredients

- 4 teaspoons olive oil
- 1 pound boneless skinless chicken breasts, cut into 1-inch cubes
- 1/2 teaspoon dried tarragon
- 1/2 teaspoon dried basil
- 1/2 teaspoon dried marjoram

- 1/2 teaspoon grated lemon zest
- 1-1/2 cups chopped carrots
- 1 cup unsweetened pineapple tidbits, drained (reserve juice)
- 1 can (8 ounces) sliced water chestnuts, drained
- 1 tart medium apple, chopped
- 1/2 cup chopped onion
- 1 cup cold water, divided
- 3 tablespoons unsweetened pineapple juice
- 3 tablespoons reduced-sodium teriyaki sauce
- 2 tablespoons cornstarch
- 3 cups hot cooked brown rice

Instructions

- In a large cast-iron or other heavy skillet, heat oil over medium heat. Add chicken, herbs and lemon zest; saute until lightly browned. Add next five ingredients. Stir in 3/4 cup water, pineapple juice and teriyaki sauce; bring to a boil. Reduce heat; simmer, covered, until chicken juices run clear and carrots are tender, 10-15 minutes.
- Combine cornstarch and remaining water. Gradually stir into chicken mixture. Bring to a boil; cook and stir until thickened, about 2 minutes. Serve with rice.

Nutrition Info

1 cup chop suey with 1/2 cup rice: 330 calories, 6g fat (1g saturated fat),

Day 29

Breakfast

Breakfast Bread Pudding

Total: 1 hr 20 min
Prep: 10 min
Inactive: 15 min
Cook: 55 min
8 servings

Ingredients

- 5 extra-large whole eggs
- 2 extra-large egg yolks
- 2 1/2 cups half-and-half
- 1/3 cup honey
- 1 1/2 teaspoons pure vanilla extract
- 2 teaspoons orange zest (2 oranges)
- 1/2 teaspoon kosher salt
- Brioche loaf
- 1/2 cup golden raisins
- Maple syrup, to serve

Instructions

- Preheat the oven to 350 degrees F.
- In a medium bowl, whisk together the whole eggs, egg yolks, half-and-half, honey, vanilla, orange zest, and salt. Set aside.
- Slice the brioche loaf into 6 (1-inch) thick pieces. Lay half brioche slices flat in a 9 by 14 by 2-inch oval baking dish. Spread the raisins on top of the brioche slices, and place the remaining slices on top. Make sure that the raisins are between the layers of brioche or they will burn while baking. Pour the egg mixture over the bread and allow to soak for 15 minutes, pressing down gently.
- Bake for 55 to 60 minutes or until the pudding puffs up and the custard is set. Remove from the oven and cool slightly before serving.

Nutrition info

Calories: 332.6
Sugars: 46.1 g
Total Carbohydrate: 53.2 g
Total Fat: 11.0 g

Lunch

Turkey Medallions with Tomato Salad

Prep: 30 min.
Cook: 15 min.
Total Time: 45 min.
6 servings

Ingredients

- 2 tablespoons olive oil
- 1 tablespoon red wine vinegar
- 1/2 teaspoon sugar
- 1/4 teaspoon dried oregano
- 1/4 teaspoon salt
- 1 medium green pepper, coarsely chopped
- 1 celery rib, coarsely chopped
- 1/4 cup chopped red onion
- 1 tablespoon thinly sliced fresh basil
- 3 medium tomatoes

TURKEY:

- 1 large egg
- 2 tablespoons lemon juice
- 1 cup panko (Japanese) bread crumbs
- 1/2 cup grated Parmesan cheese
- 1/2 cup finely chopped walnuts
- 1 teaspoon lemon-pepper seasoning
- 1 package (20 ounces) turkey breast tenderloins
- 1/4 teaspoon salt

- 1/4 teaspoon pepper
- 3 tablespoons olive oil
- Additional fresh basil

Instructions

- Whisk together first five ingredients. Stir in green pepper, celery, onion and basil. Cut tomatoes into wedges; cut wedges in half. Stir into pepper mixture.
- In a shallow bowl, whisk together egg and lemon juice. In another shallow bowl, toss bread crumbs with cheese, walnuts and lemon pepper.
- Cut tenderloins crosswise into 1-in. slices; flatten slices with a meat mallet to 1/2-in. thickness. Sprinkle with salt and pepper. Dip in egg mixture, then in crumb mixture, patting to adhere.
- In a large skillet, heat 1 tablespoon oil over medium-high heat. Add a third of the turkey; cook until golden brown, 2-3 minutes per side. Repeat twice with remaining oil and turkey. Serve with tomato mixture; sprinkle with basil.

Nutrition Info

351 calories, 21g fat (3g saturated fat), 68mg cholesterol, 458mg sodium, 13g carbohydrate (4g sugars, 2g fiber), 29g protein.

Dinner

Cod and Asparagus Bake

Prep/Total Time: 30 min.
4 servings

Ingredients

- 4 cod fillets (4 ounces each)
- 1 pound fresh thin asparagus, trimmed
- 1 pint cherry tomatoes, halved
- 2 tablespoons lemon juice
- 1-1/2 teaspoons grated lemon zest
- 1/4 cup grated Romano cheese

Instructions

- Preheat oven to 375°. Place cod and asparagus in a 15x10x1-in. baking pan brushed with oil. Add tomatoes, cut side down. Brush fish with lemon juice; sprinkle with lemon zest. Sprinkle fish and vegetables with Romano cheese. Bake until fish just begins to flake easily with a fork, about 12 minutes.
- Remove pan from oven; preheat broiler. Broil cod mixture 3-4 in. from heat until vegetables are lightly browned, 2-3 minutes.

Nutrition Info

141 calories, 3g fat (2g saturated fat), 45mg cholesterol,

Day 30

Breakfast

Sweet Millet Congee

Prep Time 10 Minutes
Cook Time 60 Minutes
Total Time:70 Minutes
Servings 8 People

Ingredients

- 1 cup Hulled Millet
- 5 cups Water
- 1 cup Sweet Potato peeled & diced
- 2 tsp Ginger minced
- 1 tsp Ground Cinnamon
- 2 Tbsp Brown Sugar
- 1 cup Apple diced
- 1/4 cup Honey
- 1 cup Bacon cooked, finely cumbled

Instructions

- Rinse and drain whole grain millet.
- Combined millet, water, sweet potato, ginger, cinnamon and brown sugar in a deep pot. Bring to a boil, reduce heat to low and simmer, stirring often, until water is absorbed, about 1 hour.
- Remove from heat and add apple, honey and bacon crumbles.

Nutrition Info

Calories: 441.9
Total Fat: 5.6 g
Cholesterol: 15.0 mg
Sodium: 191.2 mg
Total Carbs: 89.8 g

Lunch

Thai Chicken Pasta Skillet

Prep/Total Time: 30 min.
Makes
6 servings

Ingredients

- 6 ounces uncooked whole wheat spaghetti
- 2 teaspoons canola oil
- 1 package (10 ounces) fresh sugar snap peas, trimmed and cut diagonally into thin strips
- 2 cups julienned carrots (about 8 ounces)
- 2 cups shredded cooked chicken
- 1 cup Thai peanut sauce
- 1 medium cucumber, halved lengthwise, seeded and sliced diagonally
- Chopped fresh cilantro, optional

Instructions

- Cook spaghetti according to package Instructions; drain.
- Meanwhile, in a large skillet, heat oil over medium-high heat. Add snap peas and carrots; stir-fry 6-8 minutes or until crisp-tender. Add chicken, peanut sauce and spaghetti; heat through, tossing to combine.
- Transfer to a serving plate. Top with cucumber and, if desired, cilantro.

Nutrition Info

403 calories
15g fat (3g saturated fat)
42mg cholesterol
432mg sodium

43g carbohydrate

25g protein.

Dinner

Roasted Chicken Thighs with Peppers & Potatoes

Prep: 20 min.

Bake: 35 min.

Total Time: 55 min.

8 servings

Ingredients

- 2 pounds red potatoes (about 6 medium)
- 2 large sweet red peppers
- 2 large green peppers
- 2 medium onions
- 2 tablespoons olive oil, divided
- 4 teaspoons minced fresh thyme or 1-1/2 teaspoons dried thyme, divided
- 3 teaspoons minced fresh rosemary or 1 teaspoon dried rosemary, crushed, divided
- 8 boneless skinless chicken thighs (about 2 pounds)
- 1/2 teaspoon salt
- 1/4 teaspoon pepper

Instructions

- Preheat oven to 450°. Cut potatoes, peppers and onions into 1-in. pieces. Place vegetables in a roasting pan. Drizzle with 1 tablespoon oil; sprinkle with 2 teaspoons each thyme and rosemary and toss to coat. Place chicken over vegetables. Brush chicken with remaining oil; sprinkle with remaining thyme and rosemary. Sprinkle vegetables and chicken with salt and pepper.
- Roast until a thermometer inserted in chicken reads 170° and vegetables are tender, 35-40 minutes.

Nutrition Info

1 chicken thigh with 1 cup vegetables: 308 calories, 12g fat (3g saturated fat), 76mg cholesterol, 221mg sodium, 25g carbohydrate (5g sugars, 4g fiber), 24g protein. Diabetic Exchanges: 3 lean meat, 1 starch, 1 vegetable, 1/2 fat.

ANY TIME RECIPES

Grilled Tilapia with Pineapple Salsa

Prep/Total Time: 20 min.
8 servings (2 cups salsa)

Ingredients

- 2 cups cubed fresh pineapple
- 2 green onions, chopped
- 1/4 cup finely chopped green pepper
- 1/4 cup minced fresh cilantro
- 4 teaspoons plus 2 tablespoons lime juice, divided
- 1/8 teaspoon plus 1/4 teaspoon salt, divided
- Dash cayenne pepper
- 1 tablespoon canola oil
- 8 tilapia fillets (4 ounces each)
- 1/8 teaspoon pepper

Instructions

- For salsa, in a small bowl, combine pineapple, green onions, green pepper, cilantro, 4 teaspoons lime juice, 1/8 teaspoon salt and cayenne. Refrigerate until serving.
- Mix oil and remaining lime juice; drizzle over fillets. Sprinkle with pepper and remaining salt.
- Moisten a paper towel with cooking oil; using long-handled tongs, rub on grill rack to coat lightly. Grill fish, covered, over medium heat or broil 4 in. from heat 2-3 minutes on each side or until fish just begins to flake easily with a fork. Serve with salsa.

131 calories, 3g

Citrus-Herb Pork Roast

Prep: 25 min. Cook: 4 hours
8 servings

Ingredients

- 1 boneless pork sirloin roast (3 to 4 pounds)
- 1 teaspoon dried oregano
- 1/2 teaspoon ground ginger
- 1/2 teaspoon pepper
- 2 medium onions, cut into thin wedges
- 1 cup plus 3 tablespoons orange juice, divided
- 1 tablespoon sugar
- 1 tablespoon white grapefruit juice
- 1 tablespoon steak sauce
- 1 tablespoon reduced-sodium soy sauce
- 1 teaspoon grated orange zest
- 1/2 teaspoon salt
- 3 tablespoons cornstarch
- Hot cooked egg noodles
- Minced fresh oregano, optional

Instructions

- Cut roast in half. In a small bowl, combine the oregano, ginger and pepper; rub over pork. In a large nonstick skillet coated with cooking spray, brown roast on all sides. Transfer to a 4-qt. slow cooker; add onions.
- In a small bowl, combine 1 cup orange juice, sugar, grapefruit juice, steak sauce and soy sauce; pour over top. Cover and cook on low for 4-5 hours or until meat is tender. Remove meat and onions to a serving platter; keep warm.
- Skim fat from cooking juices; transfer to a small saucepan. Add orange zest and salt. Bring to a boil. Combine cornstarch and the remaining orange juice until smooth. Gradually stir into the pan. Bring to a boil; cook and stir for 2 minutes or until thickened. Serve with pork and noodles; if desired, sprinkle with fresh oregano.

Nutrition Info

5 ounces cooked pork with 2 tablespoons gravy (calculated without egg noodles): 289 calories

Veggie Cheese Soup

Prep: 15 min. Cook: 25 min.
9 servings (1-1/2 quarts)

Ingredients

- 1 medium onion, chopped
- 1 celery rib, chopped
- 2 small red potatoes, cut into 1/2-inch cubes
- 2-3/4 cups water
- 2 teaspoons reduced-sodium chicken bouillon granules
- 1 tablespoon cornstarch
- 1/4 cup cold water
- 1 can (10-3/4 ounces) reduced-fat reduced-sodium condensed cream of chicken soup, undiluted
- 3 cups frozen California-blend vegetables, thawed
- 1/2 cup chopped fully cooked lean ham
- 8 ounces reduced-fat process cheese (Velveeta), cubed

Instructions

- In a large saucepan coated with a cooking spray, cook onion and celery over medium heat until onion is tender. Stir in the potatoes, water and bouillon. Bring to a boil. Reduce heat; cover and simmer for 10 minutes.
- Combine cornstarch and cold water until smooth; gradually stir into soup. Return to a boil; cook and stir until slightly thickened, 1-2 minutes. Stir in condensed soup until blended.

- Reduce heat; add vegetables and ham. Cook and stir until vegetables are tender. Stir in cheese until melted.

Nutrition Info

115 calories, 4g fat (2g saturated fat), 15mg cholesterol, 682mg sodium, 13g carbohydrate (4g sugars, 1g fiber), 8g protein.

Thai Chicken Pasta Skillet

Prep/Total Time: 30 min.
6 servings

Ingredients

- 6 ounces uncooked whole wheat spaghetti
- 2 teaspoons canola oil
- 1 package (10 ounces) fresh sugar snap peas, trimmed and cut diagonally into thin strips
- 2 cups julienned carrots (about 8 ounces)
- 2 cups shredded cooked chicken
- 1 cup Thai peanut sauce
- 1 medium cucumber, halved lengthwise, seeded and sliced diagonally
- Chopped fresh cilantro, optional

Instructions

- Cook spaghetti according to package Instructions; drain.
- Meanwhile, in a large skillet, heat oil over medium-high heat. Add snap peas and carrots; stir-fry 6-8 minutes or until crisp-tender. Add chicken, peanut sauce and spaghetti; heat through, tossing to combine.
- Transfer to a serving plate. Top with cucumber and, if desired, cilantro.

Nutrition Info

403 calories, 15g fat (3g saturated fat), 42mg cholesterol, 432mg sodium

Italian Sausage-Stuffed Zucchini

Prep: 35 min. Bake: 20 min.
6 servings

Ingredients

- 6 medium zucchini (about 8 ounces each)
- 1 pound Italian turkey sausage links, casings removed
- 2 medium tomatoes, seeded and chopped
- 1 cup panko (Japanese) bread crumbs
- 1/3 cup grated Parmesan cheese
- 1/3 cup minced fresh parsley

- 2 tablespoons minced fresh oregano or 2 teaspoons dried oregano
- 2 tablespoons minced fresh basil or 2 teaspoons dried basil
- 1/4 teaspoon pepper
- 3/4 cup shredded part-skim mozzarella cheese
- Additional minced fresh parsley, optional

Instructions

- Preheat oven to 350°. Cut each zucchini lengthwise in half. Scoop out pulp, leaving a 1/4-in. shell; chop pulp. Place zucchini shells in a large microwave-safe dish. In batches, microwave, covered, on high 2-3 minutes or until crisp-tender.
- In a large skillet, cook sausage and zucchini pulp over medium heat 6-8 minutes or until sausage is no longer pink, breaking sausage into crumbles; drain. Stir in tomatoes, bread crumbs, Parmesan cheese, herbs and pepper. Spoon into zucchini shells.
- Place in two ungreased 13x9-in. baking dishes. Bake, covered, 15-20 minutes or until zucchini is tender. Sprinkle with mozzarella cheese. Bake, uncovered, 5-8 minutes longer or until cheese is melted. If desired, sprinkle with additional minced parsley.

Cannellini Bean Hummus

Prep/Total Time: 5 min.
1-1/4 cups (10 servings)

Ingredients

- 2 garlic cloves, peeled
- 1 can (15 ounces) cannellini beans, rinsed and drained
- 1/4 cup tahini
- 3 tablespoons lemon juice
- 1-1/2 teaspoons ground cumin
- 1/4 teaspoon salt
- 1/4 teaspoon crushed red pepper flakes
- 2 tablespoons minced fresh parsley
- Pita breads, cut into wedges
- Assorted fresh vegetables

Instructions

- Place garlic in a food processor; cover and process until minced. Add the beans, tahini, lemon juice, cumin, salt and pepper flakes; cover and process until smooth.
- Transfer to a small bowl; stir in parsley. Refrigerate until serving. Serve with pita wedges and assorted fresh vegetables.

Nutrition Info

2 tablespoons: 78 calories, 4g fat (1g saturated fat), 0 cholesterol, 114mg sodium, 8g carbohydrate (0 sugars, 2g fiber), 3g protein.

10 Shrimp Orzo with Feta

Prep/Total Time: 25 min.
4 servings

Ingredients

- 1-1/4 cups uncooked whole wheat orzo pasta
- 2 tablespoons olive oil
- 2 garlic cloves, minced
- 2 medium tomatoes, chopped
- 2 tablespoons lemon juice
- 1-1/4 pounds uncooked shrimp (26-30 per pound), peeled and deveined
- 2 tablespoons minced fresh cilantro
- 1/4 teaspoon pepper
- 1/2 cup crumbled feta cheese

Instructions

- Cook orzo according to package Instructions. Meanwhile, in a large skillet, heat oil over medium heat. Add garlic; cook and stir 1 minute. Add tomatoes and lemon juice. Bring to a boil. Stir in shrimp. Reduce heat; simmer, uncovered, 4-5 minutes or until shrimp turn pink.

- Drain orzo. Add orzo, cilantro and pepper to shrimp mixture; heat through. Sprinkle with feta cheese.

Nutrition Info

1 cup: 406 calories, 12g fat (3g saturated fat), 180mg cholesterol, 307mg sodium, 40g

Old-World Ricotta Cheesecake

Prep: 20 min. Bake: 1 hour + chilling
12 servings

Ingredients

- 1-2/3 cups zwieback, rusk or plain biscotti crumbs
- 3 tablespoons sugar
- 1/2 teaspoon ground cinnamon
- 1/3 cup butter, softened
- FILLING:
- 2 cartons (15 ounces each) ricotta cheese
- 1/2 cup sugar
- 1/2 cup half-and-half cream
- 2 tablespoons all-purpose flour
- 1 tablespoon lemon juice
- 1 teaspoon finely grated lemon zest

- 1/4 teaspoon salt
- 2 large Eggland's Best eggs, room temperature, lightly beaten
- TOPPING:
- 1 cup sour cream
- 2 tablespoons sugar
- 1 teaspoon vanilla extract

Instructions

- Combine zwieback crumbs, sugar and cinnamon; mix in butter until mixture is crumbled. Press onto bottom and 1-1/2 in. up sides of a greased 9-in. springform pan. Refrigerate until chilled.
- Preheat oven to 350°. Beat all filling ingredients except eggs until smooth. Add eggs; beat on low until combined. Pour into crust. Place pan on a baking sheet.
- Bake until center is set, about 50 minutes. Remove from oven; let stand 15 minutes, leaving oven on. Combine topping ingredients; spoon around edge of cheesecake. Carefully spread over filling. Bake 10 minutes longer. Loosen sides from pan with a knife; cool 1 hour. Refrigerate 3 hours or overnight, covering when completely cooled. Remove rim from pan. Refrigerate leftovers.

Nutrition Info

260 calories, 14g fat (9g saturated fat), 83mg cholesterol, 191mg sodium, 25g carbohydrate (16g sugars, 0 fiber), 7g protein.

Tomato Green Bean Soup

Prep: 10 min. Cook: 35 min.
9 servings

Ingredients

- 1 cup chopped onion
- 1 cup chopped carrots
- 2 teaspoons butter
- 6 cups reduced-sodium chicken or vegetable broth
- 1 pound fresh green beans, cut into 1-inch pieces
- 1 garlic clove, minced
- 3 cups diced fresh tomatoes
- 1/4 cup minced fresh basil or 1 tablespoon dried basil
- 1/2 teaspoon salt
- 1/4 teaspoon pepper

Instructions

- In a large saucepan, saute onion and carrots in butter for 5 minutes. Stir in the broth, beans and garlic; bring to a boil. Reduce heat; cover and simmer for 20 minutes or until vegetables are tender.

- Stir in the tomatoes, basil, salt and pepper. Cover and simmer 5 minutes longer.

Nutrition Info

58 calories, 1g fat (1g saturated fat), 2mg cholesterol, 535mg sodium, 10g carbohydrate (5g sugars, 3g fiber), 4g protein.

Peppered Tuna Kabobs

Prep/Total Time: 30 min.
4 servings

Ingredients

- 1/2 cup frozen corn, thawed
- 4 green onions, chopped
- 1 jalapeno pepper, seeded and chopped
- 2 tablespoons coarsely chopped fresh parsley
- 2 tablespoons lime juice
- 1 pound tuna steaks, cut into 1-inch cubes
- 1 teaspoon coarsely ground pepper
- 2 large sweet red peppers, cut into 2x1-inch pieces

- 1 medium mango, peeled and cut into 1-inch cubes

Instructions

- For salsa, in a small bowl, combine the first five ingredients; set aside.
- Rub tuna with pepper. On four metal or soaked wooden skewers, alternately thread red peppers, tuna and mango.
- Place skewers on greased grill rack. Cook, covered, over medium heat, turning occasionally, until tuna is slightly pink in center (medium-rare) and peppers are tender, 10-12 minutes. Serve with salsa.

Nutrition Info

1 kabob: 205 calories, 2g fat (0 saturated fat), 51mg cholesterol, 50mg sodium, 20g carbohydrate (12g sugars, 4g fiber), 29g protein

California Quinoa

Prep/Total Time: 30 min.
4 servings

Ingredients

- 1 tablespoon olive oil

- 1 cup quinoa, rinsed and well drained
- 2 garlic cloves, minced
- 1 medium zucchini, chopped
- 2 cups water
- 3/4 cup canned garbanzo beans or chickpeas, rinsed and drained
- 1 medium tomato, finely chopped
- 1/2 cup crumbled feta cheese
- 1/4 cup finely chopped Greek olives
- 2 tablespoons minced fresh basil
- 1/4 teaspoon pepper

Instructions

- In a large saucepan, heat oil over medium-high heat. Add quinoa and garlic; cook and stir 2-3 minutes or until quinoa is lightly browned. Stir in zucchini and water; bring to a boil. Reduce heat; simmer, covered, 12-15 minutes or until liquid is absorbed. Stir in remaining ingredients; heat through.

Nutrition Info

1 cup: 310 calories, 11g fat (3g saturated fat), 8mg

Beef and Blue Cheese Penne with Pesto

Prep/Total Time: 30 min.
4 servings

Ingredients

- 2 cups uncooked whole wheat penne pasta
- 2 beef tenderloin steaks (6 ounces each)
- 1/4 teaspoon salt
- 1/4 teaspoon pepper
- 5 ounces fresh baby spinach (about 6 cups), coarsely chopped
- 2 cups grape tomatoes, halved
- 1/3 cup prepared pesto
- 1/4 cup chopped walnuts
- 1/4 cup crumbled Gorgonzola cheese

Instructions

- Cook pasta according to package Instructions.
- Meanwhile, sprinkle steaks with salt and pepper. Grill steaks, covered, over medium heat or broil 4 in. from heat 5-7 minutes on each side or until meat reaches desired doneness (for medium-rare, a thermometer should read 135°; medium, 140°; medium-well, 145°).
- Drain pasta; transfer to a large bowl. Add spinach, tomatoes, pesto and walnuts; toss to coat. Cut steak into thin slices. Serve pasta mixture with beef; sprinkle with cheese.

Nutrition Info

532 calories, 22g fat (6g saturated fat), 50mg cholesterol, 434mg sodium, 49g carbohydrate (3g sugars, 9g fiber), 35g protein.

Mimi's Lentil Medley

Prep: 15 min. Cook: 25 min.
8 servings

Ingredients

- 1 cup dried lentils, rinsed
- 2 cups water
- 2 cups sliced fresh mushrooms
- 1 medium cucumber, cubed
- 1 medium zucchini, cubed
- 1 small red onion, chopped
- 1/2 cup chopped soft sun-dried tomato halves (not packed in oil)
- 1/2 cup rice vinegar
- 1/4 cup minced fresh mint
- 3 tablespoons olive oil
- 2 teaspoons honey
- 1 teaspoon dried basil
- 1 teaspoon dried oregano
- 4 cups fresh baby spinach, chopped
- 1 cup (4 ounces) crumbled feta cheese
- 4 bacon strips, cooked and crumbled, optional

Instructions

- Place lentils in a small saucepan. Add water; bring to a boil. Reduce heat; simmer, covered, 20-25 minutes or until tender. Drain and rinse in cold water.
- Transfer to a large bowl. Add mushrooms, cucumber, zucchini, onion and tomatoes. In a small bowl, whisk vinegar, mint, oil, honey, basil and oregano. Drizzle over lentil mixture; toss to coat. Add spinach, cheese and, if desired, bacon; toss to combine.

Nutrition Info

225 calories, 8g fat (2g saturated fat), 8mg cholesterol, 404mg sodium, 29g carbohydrate (11g sugars, 5g fiber), 10g protein

Spiced Salmon

Prep/Total Time: 20 min.
8 servings

Ingredients

- 2 tablespoons packed brown sugar
- 1 tablespoon soy sauce
- 1 tablespoon butter, melted
- 1 tablespoon olive oil
- 1/2 teaspoon garlic powder

- 1/2 teaspoon ground mustard
- 1/2 teaspoon paprika
- 1/2 teaspoon pepper
- 1/4 teaspoon dill weed
- Dash salt
- Dash dried tarragon
- Dash cayenne pepper
- 1 salmon fillet (2 pounds)

Instructions

- Mix all ingredients except salmon; brush over salmon.
- Place salmon, skin side down, on an oiled grill rack or on a lightly oiled baking sheet. Grill, covered, over medium heat or broil 4 in. from heat until fish just begins to flake easily with a fork, 10-15 minutes.

CONCLUSION

At this juncture, The D.A.S.H. Diet works to lower your blood pressure in several ways. First, by replacing high salt, highly processed foods with healthy alternatives like fruits and vegetables. A diet high in sodium has been linked to high blood pressure, which can contribute to heart disease, liver disease, kidney disease and stroke. Many sources suggest keeping your daily sodium intake to 1,500 mg per day or less. This equals about 2/3 teaspoon of salt. Use salt-free seasonings and look for salt substitutes.

DASH is also rich in nutrients such as fiber, calcium, potassium, and magnesium, deficits of which are linked to hypertension. 98% of all Americans suffer from a lack of potassium. Sources of potassium are beans, legumes, nuts, dairy products, fruits and vegetables.

The diet recommends daily servings of 7-8 of grains, 4-5 of fruits and vegetables, 2-3 of low-fat dairy, and no more than 2 of servings of lean meats. And also weekly servings of 4-5 portions of beans, seeds, and nuts.

It is easy to get to these suggested servings by making a few simple changes to your diet. You can raise your veggie intake by adding them to salads or soups, having cut or bite sized vegetables as snacks, and increasing the veggie to meat ratio in your food. You can choose whole grain versions of bread, cereal, and pasta. Add nuts into your cereal, yogurt, or salads. Have dried fruit and nuts for snacks. Substitute low-fat milk in smoothies and coffee. Use low-fat yogurt and cheese for breakfast, snacks, or on salads and vegetables.

The DASH diet is a healthy, high-fiber diet that can help, not only lower high blood pressure, but also high cholesterol. Its a healthy weight loss diet and it helps you get healthy by choosing a healthy lifestyle.